BACK PAIN? BYE BYE...!

The Best Solutions for Relief from Sciatica,
Lumbago, Slipiped Disc and Backache

Contents

Introduction

Thank you for purchasing this book. I have compiled this book with the latest knowledge about low back pain. If you suffer from low back pain or sciatica, you are not alone. About 80 percent of adults experience low back pain and 40 percent will experience sciatica in their lifetimes. Continue reading to experience a new perspective on lower back pain and sciatica!

Low back pain affects people of all ages, from the elderly to children, and is frequently the reason for medical consultations. The 2010 Global Burden Study estimates that low back pain is one of the top ten diseases and injuries that account for the highest number of disability-adjusted life years worldwide.[1] Since back pain can occur so early in life, it is difficult to estimate the incidence of first-occurrence episodes.

Lower back pain affects nearly 80 percent of all adult Americans.[2] It is not only an American problem; lower back pain is prevalent around the world. Disability caused by low back pain has risen more than 50 percent since 1990.[3] As low back pain becomes more common, the costs to patients, society, and healthcare systems continue to rise. In the United States the total costs associated with low back pain exceed $100 billion per year. Two-thirds of the total costs are attributed to lost wages and poor productivity.[4]

Sciatica affects both men and women. It is often related to another issue concerning the joints in the spine, such as herniated discs. Sciatica is not an actual diagnosis; it simply refers to pain originating from the sciatic nerve. The sciatic nerve is the longest nerve in your body. It runs from your lower back down the backside of the leg. Nerve pain is caused by inflammation or irritation to the area around the nerve.

---

[1] Damian Hoy, L. March, P. Brooks, F. Blyth, A. Woolf, C. Bain, G. Williams, E. Smith, T. Vos, J. Barendregt, C. Murray, R. Burstein, R. Buchbinder, "The global burden of low back pain: Estimates from the Global Burden of Disease 2010 study," *Annals of the Rheumatic Diseases*, 21 June 2017, vol. 73, no. 6, https://ard.bmj.com/content/73/6/968.

[2] Nadège Lemeunier, C. Leboeuf-Yde, O. Gagey, "The natural course of low back pain: A systematic critical literature review," *Chiropractic Manual Therapy*, 2012, vol. 20, p. 33.

[3] Stephanie Clark, Richard Horton, "Low back pain: A major global challenge," *The Lancet*, 9 June 2018, vol. 391, no. 10137, p. 2302, doi.org/10.1016/S0140-6736(18)30725-6.

[4] William Thomas Crow, D. R. Willis, "Estimating cost of care for patients with acute low back pain: A

retrospective review of patient records," *The Journal of the American Osteopathic Association*, April 2009, vol. 109, pp. 229-233.

PART I

THE POWERFUL MESSAGE OF PAIN

Chapter 1

The Miracle of Low Back Pain

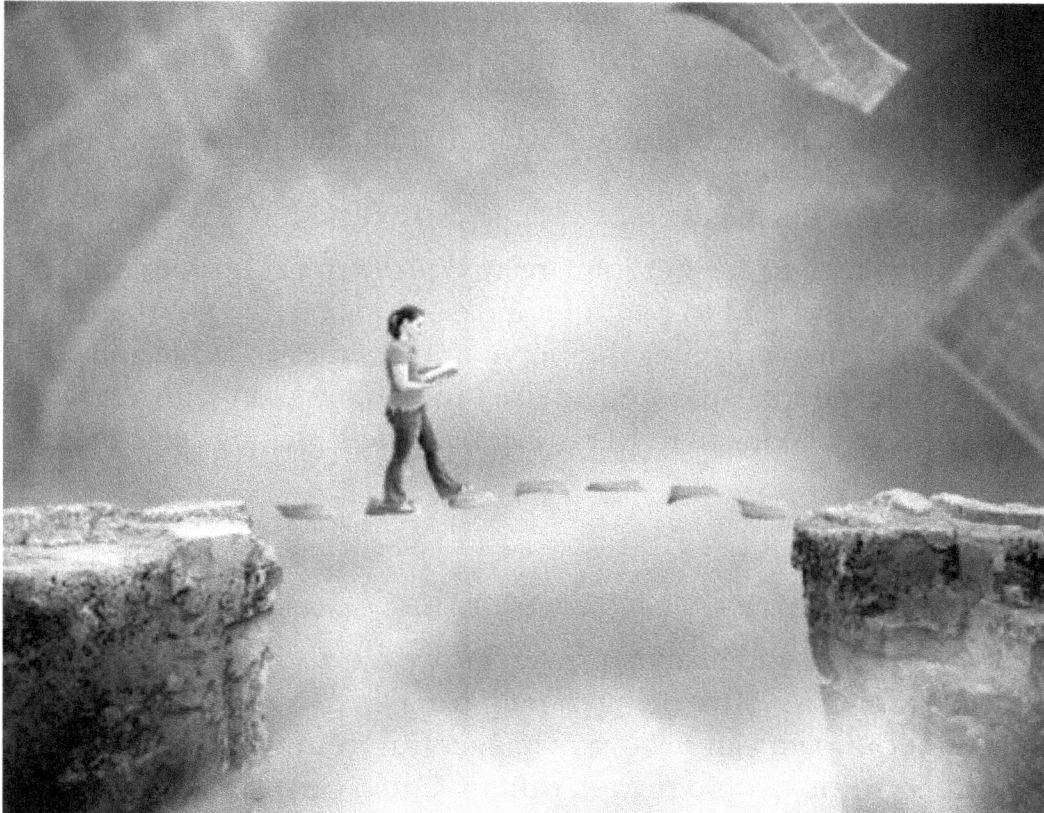

You might feel like your joint pain can't be reversed. That is a depressing thought. If you think that you have to live with it, I have great news! Not only do we have the magic wand, we can promise you that miracles can happen. That's what my patients have told me over and over again!

For example, Roberta, a forty-seven-year-old dentist with a disc protrusion in her lower back, said, "My back is in incredible pain, especially when I stand and bend over to work on my patients' teeth all day."

With my individualized program, Roberta's disc protrusion went from 11 millimeters (mm) to only 3 mm! She became pain-free and returned to work.

WHAT IS A MIRACLE?

What is a miracle? A miracle is something that happens that you can't expect or explain. It is an extraordinary event—a development or an achievement. For many people, relief from low back pain or sciatica *is* a miracle. So, where do we begin to create our own version of a miracle?

Before we continue, let's back up and take a closer look at back pain. The source of back pain can include disease, injury, age, surgery, and even stress. Any one or combination of these could be contributing factors.

Pain is often the result of less-than-optimal activity. Decreased activity can lead to faster joint deterioration. Joint deterioration occurs when muscles become weak due to age and lack of use. Once a joint loses the protection of its surrounding muscles, it can no longer tolerate the loads that result from daily activities.

Once a joint surface deteriorates, loads of daily activities become painful. Deterioration can lead to further joint-related problems. Degeneration of the spine can progress and lead to painful conditions such as spinal stenosis, disc herniation, facet joint syndrome, and nerve impingement (i.e., sciatica).

Unfortunately, people are often advised to combat pain with pain medications and reduced activity. This can become a vicious cycle that leads to more pain.

Back Pain Healing Starts With YOU!

Everybody has energy and healing power. However, some people's healing powers have decreased. After being in pain for an extended period of time, the way we think about pain can begin to change. For example, a scrape may take longer to heal in some people than in others. Often people no longer realize that they still have the ability within to reduce their pain. People have expressed feelings of depression or hopelessness. The first step to pain relief is changing how you think about pain. You don't have to be a prisoner to your pain; *you* are ready to *do* something about the pain. *You are ready to take the steps to experience pain relief!*

If you can remember to stay optimistic and embrace the fact that you DO HAVE HEALING POWER, your body will become better able to heal. You can begin to enjoy an active, pain-free lifestyle. However, remain cautious and sensible here, because you could actually hurt yourself. It is important to seek the guidance of a professional, such as a caring and compassionate physical or occupational therapist, who can empower you to become more active without causing yourself harm.

I will show you how to increase your energy and healing power.

I wish all of my clients could meet Stan. He came to my clinic with agonizing low back pain. Last year, Stan's medical doctor said, "Stan, you have arthritis in your lower back. You also have spinal stenosis and sciatica, which is likely causing the pain down your leg. I want you to see Dr. Grace Walker Gray for treatment on your back."

At his first visit Stan told me, "I am sixty-five years old. I used to be really active, but in the last two years my back has been in a lot of pain. It hurts even when walking. And getting out of the car has become increasingly difficult. I spend most of my time sitting in my lounge chair at home because of the pain."

Prolonged sitting can lead to back pain and joint deterioration. I recommended to Stan to do what most of my patients choose to do: work with me to design a holistic program to reduce his sciatica pain.

Next, we spoke about how Stan was feeling now and where he wanted to be, and we put together a program that worked for him.

When I examined Stan, I found his tight hip muscles were causing him to walk in a hunched position. I started him on a program. Do you know what step 1 was?

Step 1 for Stan's Low Back Pain

For step 1 for Stan's low back pain, I performed joint mobilization and hands-on soft tissue mobilization, gently easing the spasms in his back and buttock muscles. Spasms can compress the nerves that go down your legs. Hands-on mobilization will calm the muscles and take pressure off the legs. I applied cannabidiol oil (CBD oil) pain-relief cream along with the hands-on work.

Step 2 for Stan's Low Back Pain

For step 2, I created a program of individualized exercise for Stan. I showed him how to stretch his tight hip muscles and also gave him strengthening and core exercises to target specific muscles that support his legs during daily activities.

Step 3 for Stan's Low Back Pain

During each of Stan's visits, for step 3, I used the ML830 Laser (my magic wand) to decrease pain and inflammation and regenerate tissue.

Stan's Miracle

For Stan, his miracle came in the form of relief from his low back pain. Stan could barely drive a car before his first treatment. Today, he is back to fishing every weekend with his children and exercising at the gym. Stan was proactive in finding a solution for his problem. Miraculously, Stan is back to enjoying a pain-free life.

Chapter 2

The Dangers of Living in Pain

Have you ever considered the dangers of living in pain?

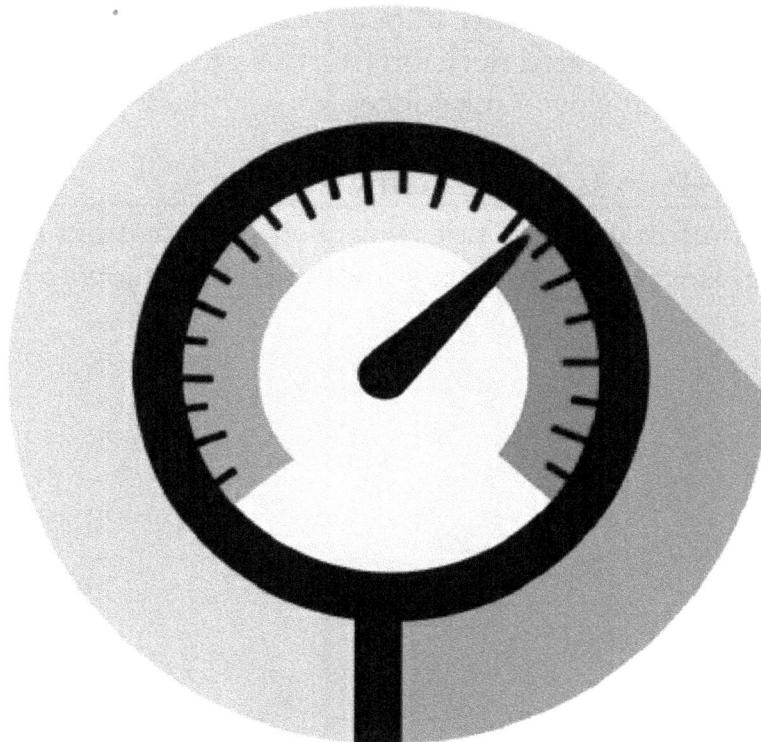

Chronic musculoskeletal pain can increase the risk of falls in older adults. A new study by a valued medical journal found that pain is directly linked to increased falls.[5] Falls are a leading cause of injury-related death and hospitalization in older adults and seniors.

Pain can affect sleep. Constant tossing and turning, whether you are asleep or not, will not allow you to enter important sleep cycles. Pain can lead to depression and in extreme cases, even suicide. Pain can even interfere with relationships at work and home.

Pain can cause anxiety and anger. Fear of the healing process and re-injury are discouraging thoughts for those living with pain.

Before Ron came to me with severe pain, he had a high-paying job in the insurance industry. He was only forty-seven when he said, "My back pain was so bad that I had to quit my job. I couldn't sit at the desk without experiencing pain. Not only did I lose my job, I felt like I lost my whole life."

Thankfully, within weeks, Ron was able to reduce his pain enough to begin working again. How? By following recommendations from me that have been outlined in this very book.

ELEVEN MISCONCEPTIONS OF BACK PAIN

If you or any of your loved ones are in pain and you're looking for somebody to help, you can make an educated decision on your next steps when you understand the following eleven misconceptions of back pain.

Misconception 1—Pain Is Your Enemy

While pain is uncomfortable, it is not your enemy. Remember that pain is natural. The brain is warning you that something is wrong with your body.

Misconception 2—You Will Need to Take Medications, Such as Painkillers and Anti-inflammatories

While medication can be a useful tool, it simply masks the pain. Deterioration and destruction will continue, although they may be less noticeable. Ask your doctor about the dangers of using prescribed and over-the-counter medication. The side effects can be shocking. Some medications can lead to complications such as liver damage and increased blood pressure. The American Heart Society recently issued a report advising doctors to recommend physical therapy for joint pain rather than prescribe medication. If your medication intake is a concern to you, speak with your doctor about alternatives.

Misconception 3—Surgery Is the Only Answer

This is untrue. Surgery should be the last resort. One patient, Joni, came to me for physical therapy after her doctor suggested this course of action. Joni said, "I wasn't ready to get on the surgery table so easily without trying other options first. I'm glad I did! Surgery is a risk I wasn't willing to take at the time."

Be vigilant; if you delay physical therapy for too long, surgery might become the only option!

Misconception 4—My Imaging Results Do Not Reflect How I Feel

Often, physicians will order X-rays, MRIs, and other tests to see if the problem might be visible. These tests can help diagnose a lot of problems. Even so, many times diagnostic procedures can lead to false positives. For instance, people can display a bulging disc but have no pain at all![6] Patients have been told their pain is coming from disc bulges or tears that look abnormal on their imaging test. Research shows that chronic back pain frequently does not reflect structural abnormalities that may appear on imaging such as MRIs. Many people with bulging discs, tears, and disc degradation are able to live pain-free and active lives.

Misconception 5—You Need to Rest Because You Are in Pain

This is not always the case—rest is not *the* solution, especially for those who are affected by chronic pain. Pain should not hold you back from reasonable activity. Often times, curtailing activity can lead to an increase in joint deterioration.

We lose muscle strength and endurance much faster than we regain it. Restricting our activity, being on work leave, or stopping our exercises deprives our bodies of physical activity for all our muscles. Taking time to let muscles recover after trauma is advisable, but long leaves from work or exercise deprive muscles of the regular activity they need in order to repair themselves. This is why muscle maintenance is so important. Muscles are able to operate at maximal efficiency when they are maintained with activity. Regular exercise likely has a preventative effect in terms of lowering the frequency of back pain and its recurrence.

Misconception 6—Low Back Pain and Sciatica Are Caused by Lifting

Lifting done incorrectly causes low back pain and sciatica. Lift with your knees, not your back or your arms. If an item is too heavy, get the help of a friend.

Misconception 7—With Low Back Pain, It Is Better to Stand Than Sit

Sitting for long periods of time puts a tremendous strain on the lower vertebrae in the spine. Many patients with sciatica report that standing is less painful. However, it is important to understand that a healthy balance of both sitting and standing is the key. Remaining in one position for an extended period of time is usually the cause of pain.

Misconception 8—If an Exercise Hurts, It Must Be Causing Harm

It is not always the case that an exercise that hurts must be causing harm. Movements that humans do every day, such as walking or standing, can cause painful elongations of the muscles. Physical therapists can work with patients to teach safe exercises for day-to-day movements.

Chronic pain can be associated with overactive nerves or pain receptors. People living with chronic pain can become very sensitive to slight, temporary pain. By understanding the difference between "harm" and "hurt," you can slowly retrain your brain to not overrespond to the pain associated with these physical activities. Even though these movements may cause more pain, this does not represent damage or harm to your spine.

Misconception 9—My Chronic Back Pain Must Be the Result of an Injury

It is possible that your chronic back pain is the result of an injury, but consider this: the human spine is capable of absorbing a phenomenal amount of energy without sustaining damage. The design of the spine is truly amazing. Some modern technological advancements have actually stemmed from its design!

By the time we develop chronic pain, our bodies may have endured several decades of wear. Acute back pain, which can occur after an injury, usually heals within six months. In a study of 1,200 people with acute back pain, less than 1 percent of participants had serious conditions. Those conditions included fractures, infections, cancers, and multiple nerve root compressions. Several treatment guidelines can identify items in your personal history or evaluation that may lead to any suspicious underlying medical conditions.

Misconception 10—There Has to Be a Perfect Treatment for Chronic Back Pain

Let's rethink this misconception of a perfect treatment for chronic back pain. Once your doctors have concluded that there is no fracture, infection, tumor, or other condition that is responsible for your pain, the next step is to look for whether there are any factors that you can use to improve your condition. Research shows that back pain is one of the top conditions to receive medical treatment in the United States. Consumers expect to be "cured" with a straightforward medication or procedure, rather than initiating their own healing response through activity.

Think back to the idea that chronic pain originates from overactive nerve or pain sensors that are amplified by the brain and spinal cord. Unfortunately, we cannot turn off your pain receptors without harming other vital functions. The correct approach is to address the root causes of your pain by focusing on muscle health and joint flexibility.

Misconception 11—It's All in Your Head

Pain is a complicated issue, involving both the mind and the body. For instance, back pain has no known cause in many cases, and stress can make it even worse. But that doesn't mean it is not real. Pain is an invisible problem that others can't see, but that doesn't mean that it's all in your head.[7]

ROBIN'S STORY

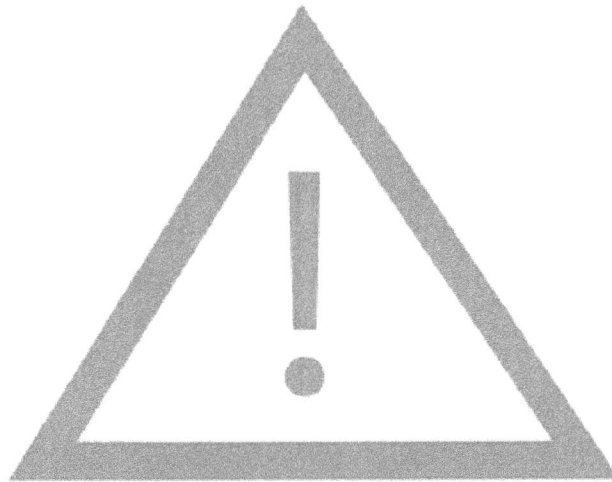

Dangerous words: "Maybe it will go away."

I want to tell you the real-life story of my friend Robin and her mother Claire. When Robin called me a year ago, there was something she wanted to tell me.

"Grace, I have terrible news. Last Christmas my mother mentioned to me that she was suffering from low back pain. I told her she needed to see you for treatment and recommendations."

I said, "Robin, I would consider it an honor to treat your mother!"

Robin then told me that her mother said, "Oh, I don't know, I think I just have to live with it. It's just wear and tear."

I asked, "Do you think she would come in for a consult with me?"

Robin replied, "I will ask her. If she agrees, I will call you."

A few months later Robin called and told me, "Grace! My mom went outside to her mailbox. When she stepped off the curb, she had a shooting pain in her back and leg. The severe pain caused her to stumble and fall. One hour later, her neighbor rushed to her side and called an ambulance. She'd fractured her hip. Grace, it's so sad. She has had a difficult time recovering at the rehab facility. I'm nervous she won't make it back to her own home."

This story is a warning. You do not have to "just deal with" pain. Spasms and shooting pain can literally bring you to your knees, and if you're not ready for it, an accident can ensue. Be proactive and find the solution for your pain rather than letting it get any worse.

The World Health Organization Recommends Prevention

According to the World Health Organization (WHO), falls are the second leading cause of death from accidental or unintentional injury worldwide.[8] Each year an estimated 646,000 individuals die from falls. Good health and strength are the best ways to avoid accidents. WHO says prevention is the best medicine!

If you have pain and aspire to live a vibrant, pain-free life with more joy and activities, work with compassionate and caring doctors, physical and occupational therapists, and/or chiropractors who specialize in pain solutions. The right healthcare professional will motivate and empower you to achieve your goals!

Be Wary Of ...

Knowledge is power. Thankfully, knowledge is at our fingertips today. *You* are your biggest advocate. It is important to educate yourself to be prepared for every professional interaction regarding your low back and sciatic pain. I've spent too much time with patients who've received ineffective treatments and misdiagnoses. I wish everyone could see the doctors that I trust, but not everyone lives in my neighborhood!

From everything I've seen in the professional world, I would like to present you with a quick list of things to consider when you are choosing a doctor or therapist.

Be Wary of Physical Therapists

Some physical therapists rely solely on their equipment to ease your pain and not on your personal ability to heal. Be wary of physical therapists who

- do not teach you something new during each visit.
- overuse modalities such as ice, heat, and electrical stimulators at the appointment and do not ask you to use ice or heat at home.
- cause more pain. If you're in more pain than when you arrived, that is unacceptable.
- only see you once and send you home with a list of exercises. That is not a skilled treatment!

Be Wary of Doctors

Be wary of doctors who

- overprescribe pain medications. After a certain amount of time, pain medication is simply a bandage. There is still an underlying injury if pain occurs without medication.
- order too many tests too soon. Diagnosis should rarely come from trial by elimination. Many MRIs discover bulging discs even though the patient is not experiencing any pain.
- push surgery. If your doctor didn't suggest physical therapy for your back pain before diving into a surgery, you should be cautious. Don't be afraid to ask to try physical therapy first. You've got nothing to lose!

If there are no red flags, there is little reason for imaging during the first four to six weeks of acute back pain. Because about 90 percent of people improve within thirty days, most well-trained doctors will not order imaging tests during an initial evaluation of acute, uncomplicated back pain. A good doctor will be knowledgeable about the therapists in the area who may be able to help you. To learn about more red flags, see chapter 3.

Be Wary of Chiropractors

Be wary of chiropractors who

- keep you coming back three times a week. I've known of people who see a chiropractor three times a week for a decade. That is just wrong! So much time and money wasted, while the core problem still exists.
- don't address the cause of your problem. Just like medications, chiropractic services can simply become a bandage.

However, understand that a good chiropractor can be helpful in treating low back pain and sciatica.

Before you choose to enter a medical clinic, physical therapy clinic, or chiropractic clinic, be sure to do your homework. Most of all—trust your gut. If you feel like your therapist or doctor is not doing everything they can for you, I encourage you to find one who will! Don't be afraid to ask for advice from friends who have medical backgrounds or are familiar with therapists and doctors in your area. Call and ask your doctor, or speak with physical therapists in the neighborhood. They will be more than happy to point you to the best doctors and chiropractors in town.

Personally, I see my chiropractor twice a month, my massage therapist once a month, and my physical therapist if I ever have an injury.

This is what David, one of my physical therapy patients, had to say: "I had just moved from Colorado when I met Dr. Grace Walker Gray at her physical therapy clinic. I had a serious pain flare-up in my low back from a car accident years ago; I needed help immediately. But I was scared—I had to see three doctors before I had any relief in the past.

"I was able to get evaluated and was recommended to a medical doctor who trusted Dr. Walker Gray. I had an MRI and X-ray taken, and was cleared to return for physical therapy with Dr. Walker Gray. Within the first week my back pain was relieved, and I haven't experienced it since!"

---

[5] Suzanne Leveille, "Chronic musculoskeletal pain and the occurrence of falls in an older population," *The Journal of the American Medical Association*, November 2009, vol. 302, no. 20, pp. 2214-2221.

[6] "Herniated disc," *MayoClinic*, 6 March 2018, https://www.mayoclinic.org/diseases-conditions/herniated-disc/symptoms-causes/syc-20354095.

[7] "Common misconceptions about chronic back pain," *University of Iowa Hospitals and Clinics*, April 2018, https://uihc.org/health-topics/common-misconceptionsabout-chronic-back-pain..

[8] "Falls prevention in older age," *World Health Organization*, https://www.who.int/ageing/projects/falls_prevention_older_age/en/.

Chapter 3

Human Anatomy and Conditions

THE VERTEBRAL COLUMN

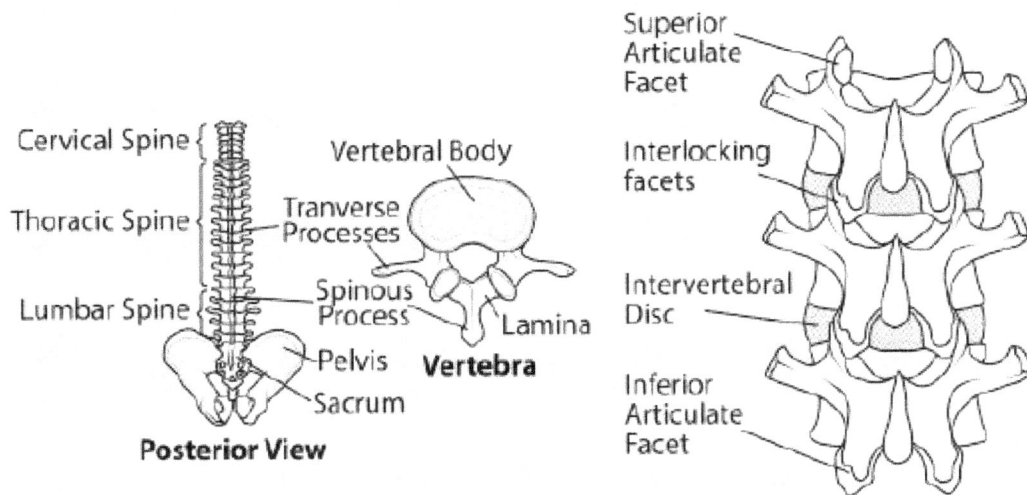

Cervical Spine
Thoracic Spine
Lumbar Spine
Pelvis
Sacrum
Posterior View

Vertebral Body
Tranverse Processes
Spinous Process
Lamina
Vertebra

Superior Articulate Facet
Interlocking facets
Intervertebral Disc
Inferior Articulate Facet

The vertebral column (a.k.a. the spine) is composed of five groups of vertebrae, beginning with seven cervical vertebrae that sit directly underneath the skull.

VERTEBRAE

Below the cervical spine are the twelve thoracic and five lumbar vertebrae. Even lower are the sacrum and coccyx, fused together. Each vertebra contains facets that resemble gears, or grooves, that fit each other. These facets allow the spine to bend and twist as one while maintaining structural integrity to protect the spinal cord.

Discs

A healthy vertebral column includes soft discs to help cushion the space between each vertebra. Vertebral discs are soft, cushiony pads that act as shock absorbers within the spine. They are located between one vertebra and the next.

As we age, our vertebral discs can become thin and weak.

Weak discs can cause lower back pain, leg pain, and other symptoms such as numbness and weakness. Disc herniation occurs when the fluid within the discs protrudes out of the disc and presses on surrounding tissue. This protrusion can lead to nerve impingements. More on this will be discussed below in "Conditions of the Low Back."

Spinal Cord

Inside the strong, bony vertebral column is the fragile spinal cord. This structure contains nerves that originate in the brain. The spinal cord runs from the brain stem all the way to the bottom of the spine. The spinal cord is one of the most important parts of your body. It is the main relay between your mind and body; each movement is transferred from your brain to your body via an instruction, and every sensation travels from your body to your brain through the spinal cord.

Nerves

The nerves are amazing structures. Nerves are special cells that vary in length. Some are very long, to allow them to transfer messages long distances very fast —fast enough for you to react to a foul ball or avoid a car accident. There are two types of nerves, also known as *neurons*. One set is responsible for sending signals to muscles to produce movement (motor neurons), and the other sends sensory signals—such as hot, cold, pain, and so on—to the brain (sensory neurons).

The nerves are the body's all-natural electrical cords, constantly cycling in sensory information ("the plate is hot") and relaying back a motor response ("move your hand"). Radiculopathy is a condition that affects the nerves. It is caused by compression, inflammation, or injury to a nerve root. Pressure on the nerve root can cause pain, numbness, and tingling that affects the immediate area and can radiate to other parts of the body as well.

Muscles

Groups of muscles that surround joints work together to produce movements. Muscles only work in one direction, and they are either contracting or relaxing. For instance, when you bend your arm at the elbow, one group of muscles pulls in only one direction. When you straighten your arm at the elbow, the first set of muscles (called the *agonist* group) relaxes, while the opposite muscle group (*antagonist*) contracts to perform the movement.

Since there are always at least two sets of muscles to counteract each other and create balance, things begin to get tricky. For example, if a group of muscles on one side of the spine is stronger than the ones on the opposite side, bad posture may develop.

Conditions of the Low Back

It is very difficult to perform surgery for spinal pain, due to the delicacy and intricacy of the components of the vertebral column. While the functions the spine performs are amazing, they pose a serious concern regarding surgery. Many diagnoses, such as degenerative discs, cannot be cured. Instead, special exercise programs and precautions can severely slow the process of degeneration. Pinched nerves can be relieved by reducing inflammation around the area. Inflammation plays a big role in pain that originates from the spine.

Inflammation is painful because everything in the surrounding area is under an unusual amount of pressure from the incoming blood and lymph. If we can reduce inflammation to an area, we can likely reduce pain as well. Once inflammation reduction is followed by strengthening exercises, we have a good foundation for preventing pain in the future.

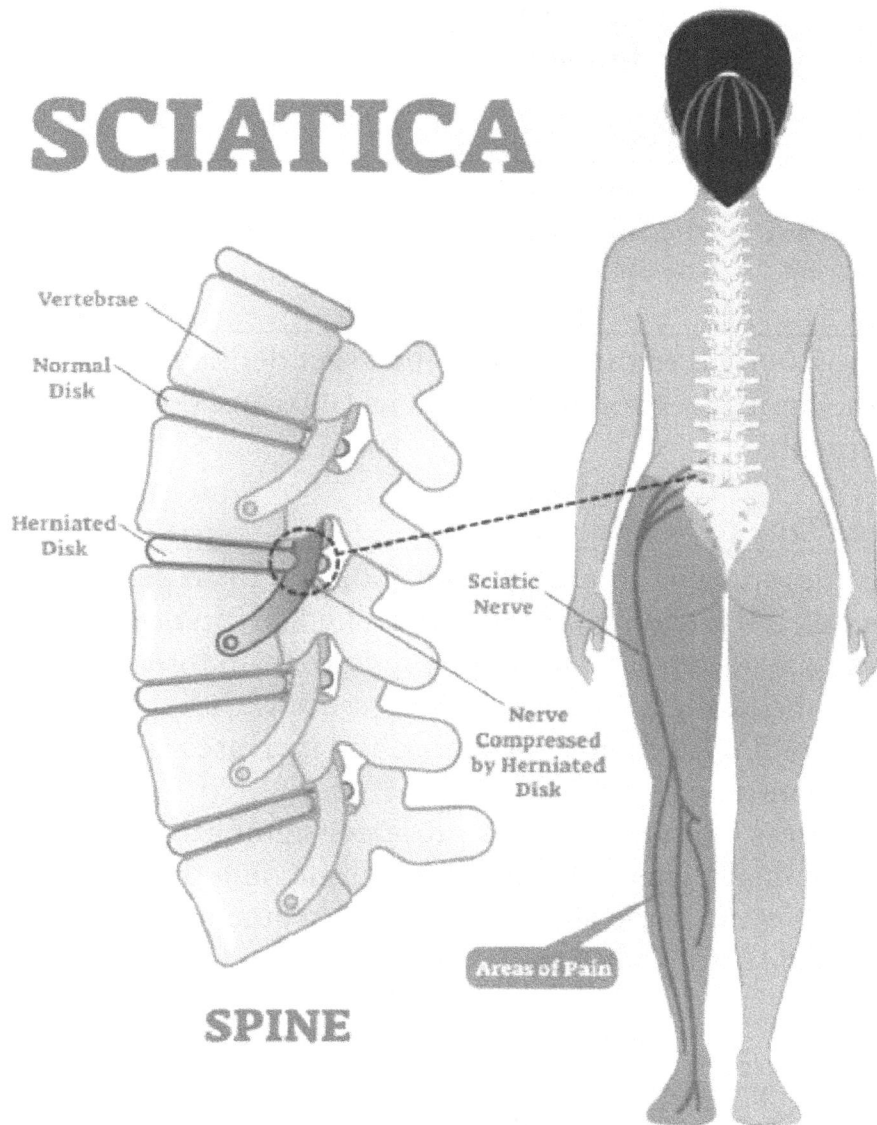

SCIATICA

Vertebrae

Normal Disk

Herniated Disk

Sciatic Nerve

Nerve Compressed by Herniated Disk

Areas of Pain

SPINE

Sciatica

Sciatica is actually the inflammation of the sciatic nerve. The nerve runs from the lumbar spine, around the hips, and down the backside of your leg. It is the longest nerve in the body. Sciatica can occur due to conditions that affect the spine, such as a herniated or degenerative disc, by putting the sciatic nerve under increased pressure.

Low Back Pain

The most common joint pain people experience is low back pain, also known as *lumbago*. In people over forty-five, the most common cause of low back pain is degeneration of the joints and discs. Low back pain is a general diagnosis that can include many conditions, such as disc herniation, nerve impingement, spinal stenosis, and facet joint syndrome.

Lumbago

The term *lumbago* is most often used by doctors and pain specialists. Lumbago simply refers to pain in the muscles and joints of the lower back.

Backache

Backache is a loosely used term; however, the exact definition refers to a pain, especially in the lumbar region of the back, usually caused by the strain of a muscle or ligament.

Bulging Discs Due to Weakness

Discs between the spinal cord are composed of two main parts: a series of leathery rings called the *annulus fibrosus* and a jelly-like interior named the *nucleus pulposus*. During day-to-day activities, the pressure from movements inside the nucleus stresses the leathery exterior. The pressure within the nucleus actually doubles when standing compared to sitting, and increases sixfold during a forward-bending motion.

As we age, stress from the nucleus produces significant wear and tear on the annulus. The annulus begins to have trouble containing the nucleus, which is how the term *bulging disc* came about. The entire segment becomes unstable, and can produce spinal stiffness and pain.

Prolapsed Disc

When the annulus within the disc begins to break down, a tear or channel can cause the nucleus to bulge outside the disc. Worse yet, the nucleus can actually squeeze out from the center of the disc. This severe condition is known as a disc herniation, or prolapsed disc.

A prolapsed disc can lead to a violent inflammatory reaction. Some people have said it feels as though they were stabbed with a knife in their spine. This pain is due to the body attacking the nucleus with infection-fighting cells because it does not recognize the nucleus in that location. It's the body's way of telling you that something is (really) wrong!

Slipped Disc

The term *slipped disc* is often misused. The exact definition concerns a vertebral disc that is displaced or partly protruding, pressing on nearby nerves and causing back pain or sciatica.

Spondylosis

The medical term for a stiff vertebral column is *spondylosis*. Spondylosis is common for middle-aged adults. It develops when the annulus is subjected to repetitive microtrauma (small injuries). As we go through life, the annulus heals itself from these small tears with scar tissue. Because scar tissue is not as flexible as the typical annulus fibers, the disc becomes stiffer. After this cycle repeats many times, the annulus becomes so stiff that it becomes inflexible. Consequently, the lower back joints become painful to move.

Ligament Sprains

As with all joints in your body, your spine is held together with strong fibrous ligaments. As we go through life and subject our bodies to stress and trauma, our ligaments begin to degrade and can tear. It might be helpful for you to know that ligaments are subject to *sprains*, whereas muscles experience *strains*.

Ligament tears are classified by three grade levels. A grade 1 tear means that the fibers have experienced some sprain but are intact. A grade 2 sprain means the fibers experienced significant sprain but are intact. A grade 3 sprain means the ligament experienced such a significant sprain that the ligament completely tore. Often times, a severe tear (grade 2) is more painful than a complete tear (grade 3).

When you sprain your back, as with most injuries, inflammation begins to develop. Inflammation around the spine is not always visible; even the slightest amount of inflammation can put a tremendous amount of pressure between the tight tolerances between vertebrae. Ligament sprains can cause your back to become either stiff or unstable, depending on whether your ligament is still attached. Ligament sprains require a specialized approach to treatment, depending on their severity.

Coccyxdynia

Coccyxdynia specifically refers to a sprain in the ligaments that hold the coccyx to the sacrum. Normally, there is very little movement between these bones. There is usually, however, a small amount of flex between them, which allows for some shock absorption, but that is all. There is only one way you can sprain these ligaments: a serious fall resulting in your landing on your bottom. Most of the pain from this type of sprain leads to—you guessed it—swelling. However, movement of this joint can cause very painful sprains, due to the large nerves that pass through the area and down to the legs.

Additionally, women with children may be susceptible to increased complications in this area. The ligaments in this area, which are normally fused, allow more movement in women in the final stages of pregnancy. This can lead to further joint complications.

Arthritis

Arthritis is common for many people as we age. There are over 150 types of arthritis; some are autoimmune and others develop over time. This text refers to one of the most common forms, osteoarthritis.

Everyone has some degree of arthritis. Arthritis usually develops more rapidly in areas that have been injured or have experienced trauma. Arthritis is simply the wear and tear of a joint, which causes inflammation.

Arthritis care can be difficult because joints become inflamed with overuse. Many people decide to stay away from exercise if they suffer from arthritis. However, exercise to strengthen muscles and maintain joint flexibility is essential to prevent flare-ups from occurring during normal movement. Tricky, isn't it? The key is to find the right amount of preventative exercise without overdoing it. For most who attempt to exercise without help from a professional, it is a trial-and-error experience.

Displaced Vertebra

A displaced vertebra (also known as *spondylolisthesis*) usually occurs with the lower lumbar vertebrae. A vertebra can slide out of alignment over time. Many people can go on living their normal lives, and even play rigorous sports, without knowing their spine is out of alignment. This displacement is not sudden, nor is it accompanied by pain, cracking, or any other sensation.

The bones themselves do not hurt; however, the adjacent discs and facet joints begin to rapidly degrade, which can lead to pain stemming from disc damage. Displaced bones only occur for a few reasons, such as birth defects and severe degeneration.

Nerve Root Compression

When a severe disc injury occurs, the nucleus of the disc can push on one of the many nerve roots in the spine. The nerve root that is closest to the disc is the motor neuron. It carries signals to the muscles. If a nerve root is badly compressed, it can affect your strength and ability to control movements in the legs and feet, for instance.

When a sudden onset of lower body weakness occurs, a doctor may consider if a back injury is the culprit. Thankfully, the nerve root that carries sensory signals to the brain (the sensory neuron) is further away from the disc, in the spinal canal. It is less common for a disc to protrude so far that it reaches these sensory nerves. If protrusions were to reach that far, you can bet it would be extremely painful!

BACK PAIN: RED FLAGS

When is it time to schedule a doctor's appointment? If your back pain is starting to affect your normal life because of disruptions to work or sleep, then it is time. There are several red flags to become familiar with. The purpose of these warning signs is to detect fractures, infections, or tumors of the spine. If you are experiencing one or more of the red flags listed below, schedule an appointment with your doctor as soon as possible.

Fever

While it is possible your back pain is being caused by a fever, it is also possible that it could be a warning sign of a more serious systemic condition. If it is just an infection, simple antibiotics can normally alleviate the problem. Most doctors recommend you slowly return to your daily activities once you start to feel better.

Trauma

If you have had a traumatic event recently—such as a fall or car accident—your doctor will want to take a serious look at your back pain. Even a minor fall, when you are older, can cause a fracture. Expect the doctor to take an X-ray to rule out any fractures. Your pain may be managed with medication and eventually a referral to a physical therapist.

Numbness and Tingling

You might think you can alleviate tingling and numbness with over-the-counter medication, but such symptoms usually indicate inflammation or nerve irritation. Nerve pain can be more significant than a typical pain. If numbness and tingling persist, it could mean that you are experiencing one of several conditions, such as a herniated disc or spinal stenosis. Untreated nerve damage can lead to permanent disabilities.

Loss of Bowel Function

Loss of bowel or bladder control, coupled with back pain, could be a telltale sign of a rare but serious condition named *cauda equina syndrome*. This syndrome occurs when the nerve roots in the lower end of the spinal cord have experienced a compression and become unable to function. This can be the result of a herniated disc, fracture, tumor, trauma, or spinal stenosis. Symptoms include numbness and weakness of the legs. Cauda equina syndrome is a medical emergency that requires immediate medical attention. Your doctor can perform a procedure called a *surgical decompression* to relieve your pain.

History of Cancer, Immune System Suppression, Osteoporosis, or Chronic Steroid Use

If you have a history of cancer, it is important for the doctor to rule out the possibility that the cancer has spread to your back. Immune-system suppression could lead your doctor to suspect an infection as the cause of your back pain. A history of osteoporosis or chronic steroid use could help your doctor to identify a fracture as the cause of your pain.

Foot Drop

If you find it difficult to raise your toes when you are walking, causing them to drag, you may be experiencing *foot drop*. Foot drop normally happens on only one side of the body. It is typically the sign of a greater issue, usually a nerve problem that occurs when the nerve that activates the muscles to lift your foot when you walk is not working properly. A doctor is needed to figure out the cause of your foot drop, and may suggest physical therapy or steroid injections.

Prolonged Pain

Pain that is prolonged for more than six weeks is a red flag, as 90 percent of back pain cases get better within six weeks. It is important for your doctor to know how long you have been in pain, to determine whether or not it is chronic. Your doctor will want to investigate more serious underlying causes if your pain is still severe after six weeks. Expect more in-depth blood work and imaging tests to be conducted to help determine a diagnosis.

Unexplained Weight Loss

If you have been experiencing unexplained weight loss, your doctor should be aware of it in order to rule out infection or tumors as possible causes for your back pain. Doctors may order blood work or an MRI to check for infection or tumors.

TESTS

X-rays

X-rays of the whole spine, neck, upper back, or lower back may be performed to diagnose the cause of back pain—fractures (broken bones), arthritis, spondylolisthesis, degeneration of the discs, tumors—or abnormalities in the curvature of the spine, such as a kyphosis (rounded upper back) or a scoliosis (a sideways curve).

MRIs

An MRI scan provides a different type of image from other tests such as X-rays or ultrasounds. An MRI of the lumbar spine shows the bones, discs, spinal cord, and the spaces through which nerves pass between the vertebral bones. An MRI can detect a variety of conditions of the lumbar spine, including problems with the bones (vertebrae) or the soft tissues (spinal cord, nerves, and discs). It can assess the discs to see whether or not they are bulging, ruptured, or pressing on the spinal cord or nerves.

Electromyogram

An electromyogram (also known as an EMG) is a test that involves placing very small needles into the muscles to monitor electrical activity. It is normally reserved for more chronic pain, to help identify the level of nerve root damage. This test is also able to help the doctor distinguish between nerve root disease and muscle disease.

CT Scans

CT scans (commonly called CAT scans) are X-rays that produce cross-sectional pictures of a specific part of the body. The scanning machine circles the body in order to produce a three-dimensional picture, providing greater detail. During this type of procedure, your doctor will inject a contrast dye into your bloodstream. The dye allows the machine to take clear pictures of your blood vessels and organs. CT scans usually take thirty to forty-five minutes and have very few risks.

PART II

RELIEF FROM SCIATICA, LUMBAGO, SLIPPED DISC, AND BACKACHE

Chapter 4

Solution One: Five Do's and Four Don'ts

"My back is out!! Now what do I do?"

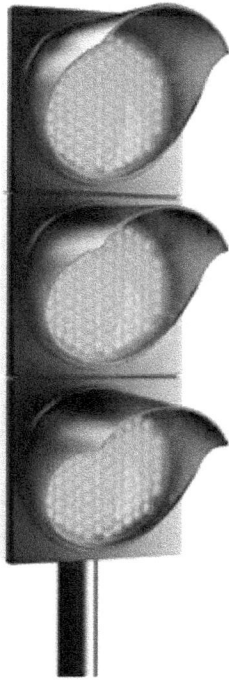

Green Light

One of the most confusing things for someone experiencing sciatica or low back pain is determining when to use heat and when to use ice. Generally, ice is preferable when the issue is caused by a nerve compression. Heat is more effective for reducing muscle contractions associated with sciatica. We have already discussed various thoughts about determining the cause of your symptoms, but when in doubt, refer to this simple guideline to help determine when to use heat and when to use ice.

If you have sharp, intense, or "electric" feelings of pain, with or without swelling, this usually indicates there is inflammation present. Inflammation is treated with ice.

In contrast, if your symptoms are mostly stiffness or mild soreness, there is usually no inflammation present. In this situation, heat is a better option. A generic heat pack from your favorite online or retail store will do. Please be cautious of burns the first time you use it. Although heat may feel good, it does increase the inflammatory response of the body. Ultimately, you could be causing more pain and inflammation. Please err on the side of caution when using a hot pack.

With regard to treating low back pain and sciatica, I always recommend starting with ice. Most people respond better to it. A smaller percentage of people do respond better to heat, no matter what science tells us should and should not work. It is important for you to find that out for yourself; however, I recommend starting with ice.

1. Do Use Ice

Ice is a natural anti-inflammatory. Many people today associate its use with the reduction of painful inflammation.

Inflammation can be difficult to treat. It is not uncommon for it to come in cycles. Perhaps you have experienced the feeling from an accident long ago, much as has my client Dave.

"Years ago, I strained my low back. I experienced painful inflammation, but X-rays and MRIs came back with no problems. Ever since, I have become prone to straining the same area in my back. I sacrificed my leisure life to make sure I could save my back and keep working."

Dave was in pretty bad shape when I saw him. His fear kept him from enjoying life. His problem was that he was unable to maintain himself at home by simply using ice. After careful instruction on how and when to use ice, he was able to regain his leisure lifestyle. He returned to fishing and I haven't heard back from him since his consultation.

What was the secret he used at home to relieve painful inflammation? A little secret that I learned from www.military.com is that there is a jewel hiding in my cupboard: popcorn. Yes, popcorn.[9]

Unpopped popcorn kernels in bags make fantastic cold packs. They are inexpensive, reusable, and very efficient. They are able to retain cold for a very long time without ever getting too cold. If you find your cold pack is too cold, a paper towel will make it tolerable.

While some cold packs can be uncomfortable and get soggy, bags of popcorn kernels stay dry. When weight is uncomfortable, another advantage is that they also do not weigh much.

Most back pain is accompanied by some type of inflammation, and addressing the inflammation helps reduce the pain. Ice numbs sore tissues, providing pain relief similar to a local anesthetic. Icing even decreases tissue damage. A massage adds the beneficial effects of gentle manipulation of the soft tissues. Use ice for ten minutes twice a day—once in the morning and then once just before you go to sleep.

2. Do Use Heat

Although using hot packs can initiate an inflammatory response, some people do find more relief from heat. If you want to save money and not buy reusable or one-use, I suggest using a hot water bottle wrapped in a towel to target specific areas, or using an electrical moist heat pack. If your lower back is bothering you, try placing the heat pack behind your back while you sit in a chair. Besides watching for burns, be sure to use heat for no more than fifteen minutes. I have had several patients fall asleep while they were self-administering heat. Please be careful!

Warm baths are also an effective way to administer heat, but the same warning applies. Heat can cause an inflammatory response. If you have had inflammation in parts of your body for an extended amount of time and you are the type of person who takes a hot bath every night, you might want to rethink your approach!

3. Do Utilize Your Abdominal Muscles During Activity

Pull your tummy in for all exertion. This activates your core abdominal muscles, which are responsible for stabilizing your lower back. Not utilizing your abdominal muscles during activity is one of the most common mistakes people make as they age. It is easy to become reliant on the stronger posterior muscles that make up your backside. This creates a strength imbalance around the spine, which is why it is so important to practice your exercises often. Your abdominal muscles are there to help your back. Train them! Use them! And remember, when your back goes into spasm, your core abdominal muscles reflexively let go! You need to train them to work again to support your low back.

4. Do Put Pillows under Your Knees When Lying on Your Back

When you are lying on your back for any reason, put pillows under your knees. If you're a side sleeper, a pillow between your knees will help to relieve pressure in your low back and hips. Your body has a natural curve that does a very good job at supporting itself in the upright position. However, many people pay little attention to the area in the lumbar spine that naturally rises off the mattress when we lie flat on our backs. To relieve pressure in this area, be sure to place a pillow under your knees when you are sleeping.

Keep reading for more sleeping information in the posture section in "Chapter 6: Solution Three."

5. Do Your Exercises Twice Each Day

See the next chapter for the top twelve exercises to reduce sciatica and low back pain.

See "Chapter 6: Solution Three" for more advice on daily activities.

FOUR DON'TS

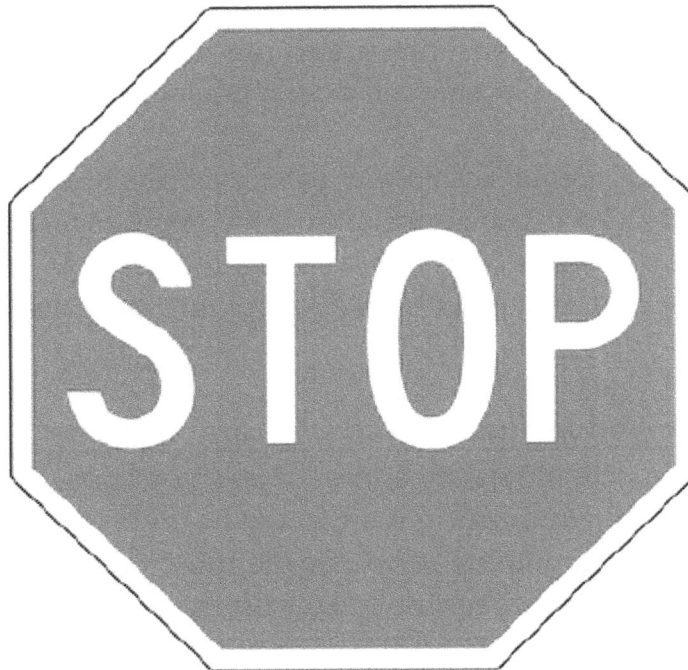

1. Don't Sit for More Than Twenty Minutes at a Time

Sitting for prolonged periods of time is one of the worst things you can do for your sciatica and low back pain. Circulation can become limited when sitting. In addition, most people sit in un-ergonomic positions. Be sure you get up and walk around the home or office, go to the bathroom, or grab a drink of water once every twenty minutes. Even when you are sitting in your comfortable recliner, you are subject to this rule.

2. Don't Lift More Than Ten Pounds at a Time and Use Your Knees

Don't lift more than 10 lb. at a time, and bend with your knees. This is extremely important for anyone who is recovering from sciatica or low back pain. In fact, this is one of the most important precautions that doctors and physical therapists set for everyone who is being treated for sciatica or low back pain.

Be cautious of your body, and listen to what it is telling you. Work smarter, not harder. Be sure to bend with your knees when lifting objects, and avoid movements that involve bending or twisting.

3. Don't Twist

Avoid twisting motions, especially while lifting. Bending and twisting is extraordinarily hard on your back. Ligaments that stabilize the spine must work their hardest to maintain stability when the spine twists.

4. Don't Jump Out of Bed

Be mindful about how you are getting out of bed. Muscles are most relaxed after sleeping and they haven't had a chance to warm up. Use the "log roll" techniques to roll to one side of the bed without bending your back. Next, use your hands and arms to slowly push yourself up to sit on the edge of the bed. Lastly, use leg (not back or arm) strength to stand up.

---

[9] "Random tip of the day: Ice packs," *Military.com*, 3 June 2010, https://www.military.com/paycheck-chronicles/2010/06/03/random-tip-of-the-day-ice-packs.

Chapter 5

Solution Two: Exercise

TOP TWELVE EXERCISES

There are many studies in the literature showing how core and lumbar-stabilization exercises are effective in alleviating low back pain.[10]

In fact, according to the National Institute of Neurological Disorders and Stroke, "exercise may be the most effective way to speed recovery from low back pain and help strengthen back and abdominal muscles."

Home exercises are usually prescribed at the beginning of physical therapy and modified throughout the course of care. They are provided to reinforce progress that is made during treatment and are intended to be used continuously after therapy to maintain health and performance. I find that clients who are compliant with their home exercise programs make tremendous progress.

If there are two mistakes that people make most often when practicing exercises, they are (1) they are not breathing, and (2) they are attempting the exercises without using supporting muscles.

Be sure you are engaging the appropriate supporting muscles, such as the ones in your abdomen and backside. These are the core muscles that were referenced previously. Too often people hurt themselves trying to complete exercises by compensating with the incorrect muscles. If something is causing any irregular pain, stop immediately. Always check with your doctor or physical therapist before attempting new exercises.

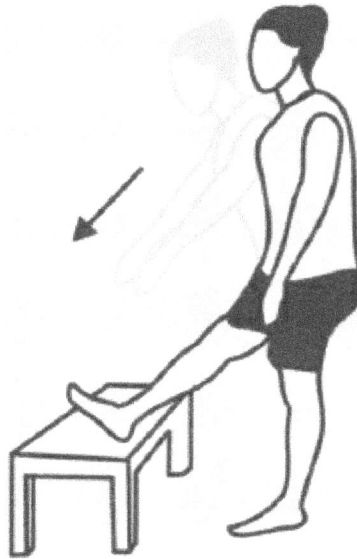

Figure 1: Standing Hamstring Strech

Exercise 1: Standing Hamstring Stretch

Your hamstring muscles are located in the back of your thighs. This group of muscles starts in the hips and runs down the back of the leg to connect just above the calf. When these muscles contract, your hip and knee bend. Tight hamstrings are a common complaint, especially for people who play sports.

1. Begin this exercise standing in front of a surface raised between 4 and 12 inches.
2. Place the heel of one foot on the raised surface.
3. Extended the toes on that foot so they begin to point upwards, slightly. Extend the knee so your leg is straight.
4. Slowly reach both arms toward your toes. You will start to feel the stretch behind your knee and up to your hips.
5. Hold a comfortable stretch for 10 seconds.
6. Repeat 10 times with each leg.
7. This stretch can also be done seated on the ground on a yoga mat with leg extended comfortably in front of you.

Exercise 2: Gluteal Stretch

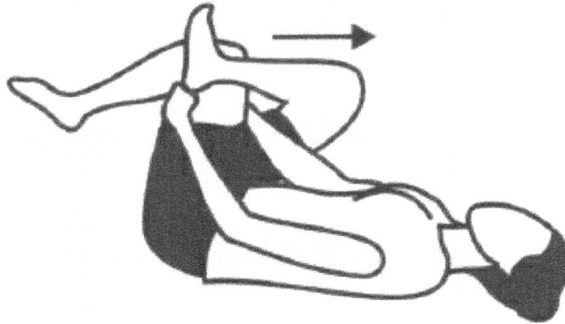

Figure 2: Gluteal Strech

The gluteal muscles comprise three major muscles that make up the buttocks, which assist us in standing from a seated position, climbing stairs, and staying in an erect position. Consult your doctor before attempting this movement, as it may not be recommended for those with hip replacements.

1. Start on your back with your palms facedown by your hips. Keep your feet flat and knees bent.
2. Bring one leg up and cross it over the other, with your ankle resting above the knee of your supporting leg.
3. Grab behind the knee of your supporting leg and pull it straight to your chest.
4. Hold this position for 10 seconds.
5. Repeat 10 times on each leg.

Exercise 3: Hip Flexor Stretch

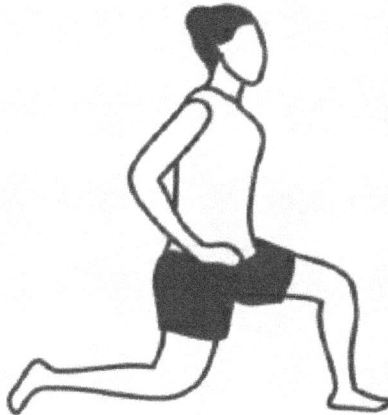

Figure 3: Hip Flexor Strech

The hip flexors are located on the front of your thighs. Their job is to flex, or bend, the hip to allow you to raise your foot up from the floor to walk or perform other movements.

Begin this stretch in a standing position. Use a solid surface to support yourself with your hand if need be.

1. Take one step forward to have a comfortable distance (between 18 and 24 inches) between your front and back foot.
2. Slowly lower your trailing knee (whichever knee is in back) down to the floor to begin the stretch.
3. Hold this position for 10 seconds.
4. Repeat 10 times with each leg.

Exercise 4: ISO-Abs

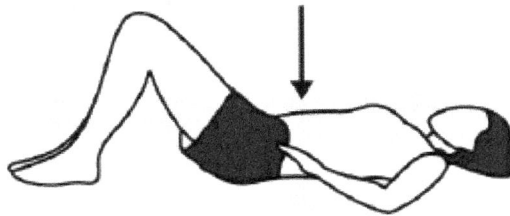

Figure 4: ISO Abs

The term *ISO* refers to "isometric muscle contractions." Isometric contractions occur when there is a muscle contraction without actual movement. When your back goes into spasm, your core abdominal muscles let go and cease to support your back. It is essential that the abdominal muscles are exercised. Coordinate this activity with breathing.

1. Lie on your back comfortably with your legs bent and the soles of your feet flat on the ground.
2. As you slowly exhale from your mouth, suck your tummy in.
3. Breathe in through your nose, and let your abdomen expand.
4. Repeat 10 times.

Exercise 5: Pelvic Tilt

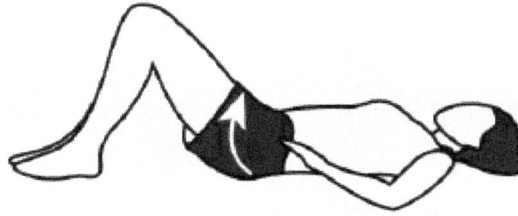

Figure 5: Pelvic Tilt

There are many ways to develop strong abdominal core muscles besides performing sit-ups. The pelvic tilt is a fantastic way to exercise the same abdominal muscles with less strain on your neck and back.

1. Begin lying faceup on a yoga mat, floor, or stable surface.
2. Place your arms comfortably at your sides.
3. Place the soles of your feet flat on the floor with your knees bent. Engage your abdominal and gluteal (buttock) muscles. Lift your bottom up off the ground.
4. Keep your spine straight.
5. Hold this position for 10 seconds.
6. Repeat 10 times.

Exercise 6: Lumbar Extension

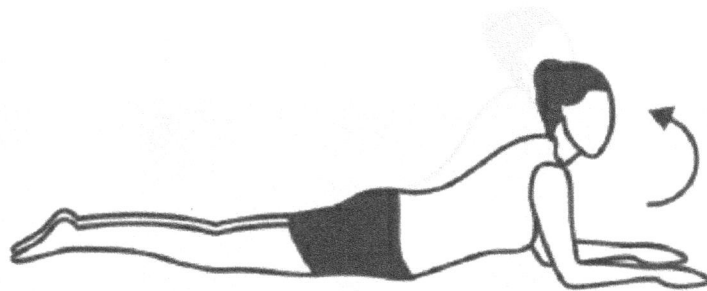

Figure 6: Extension Exercise

It is important to perform extension stretches alongside spine flexion exercises to focus on both muscle groups that act on the spine. The lumbar spine can be stretched without putting much strain on the rest of the body. (However, if you have been diagnosed with a spondylolisthesis, do not do this exercise.)

1. Begin facedown, as if you were preparing to do an ISO-abs exercise.
2. Place your palms flat on the floor in front of your shoulders.
3. Push up with your arms into a half push-up, but do not lift your hips.
4. Hold this position for 10 seconds.
5. Repeat 10 times.

Exercise 7: Planks

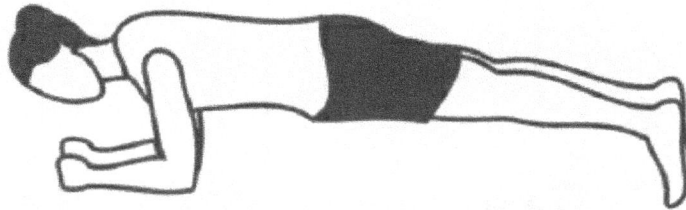

Figure 7: Elbow Plank

Once you feel comfortable performing the ISO-abs and pelvic tilt exercises, planks are a good upgrade. Planks are very useful exercises for building core abdominal strength.

1. Begin facedown on a yoga mat, floor, or stable surface (not a mattress or couch).
2. Place your palms flat on the floor by your head with your forearms and elbows flat, as if you were going to do a push-up.
3. With your toes firmly tucked in and planted, engage your abdominal muscles and bring your body up off the ground in a push-up position from the elbows.
4. Be sure your abdomen is tight and your back is straight.
5. Hold this position for 10 seconds.
6. Repeat 10 times.

Exercise 8: Sit to Stand

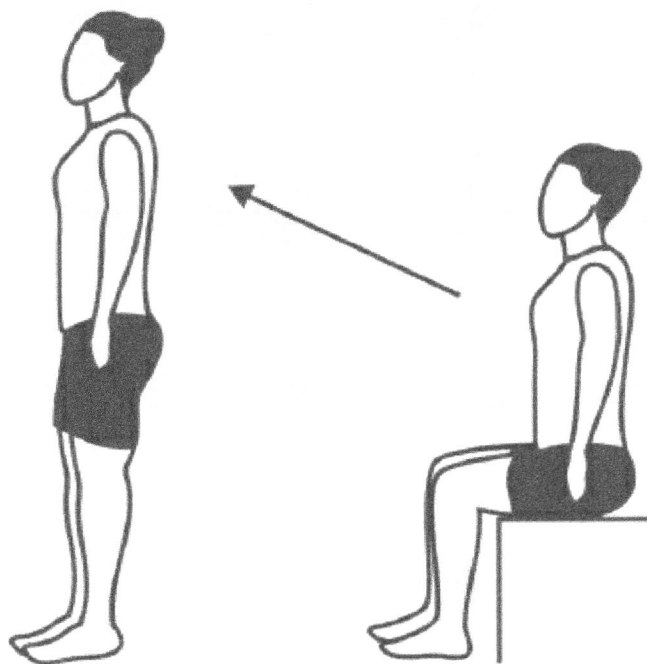

Figure 8: Sit to Stand

Multiple times a day many people perform sit-to-stand activities, such as getting up from a car or chair. However, it would be wise to practice this movement while maintaining proper posture and body mechanics, by using leg power to stand rather than using your back. Remember not to push up from the seating surface with the hands or arms in this exercise—focus on leg strength.

1. Begin sitting in a chair with your feet flat on the floor and knees bent at 90 degrees.
2. Place your arms comfortably at your sides.
3. Engage abdominal and buttock muscles and stand straight up, limiting the engagement of the back muscles.
4. Sit back down slowly, without "plopping" down.
5. Repeat 10 times.

Exercise 9: Bridge

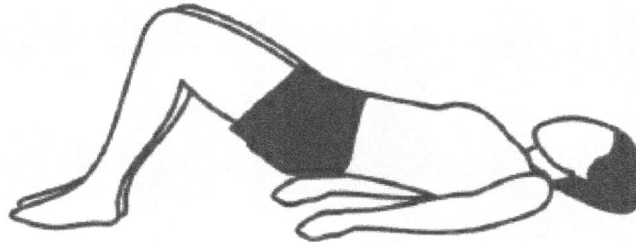

Figure 9: Bridge

Bridging is a great exercise to strengthen your gluteal muscles and hamstrings. Begin on your back on a yoga mat.

1. Have your feet flat on the mat and your knees bent. Rest your palms on the mat at your side, comfortably.
2. Breathe in. As you exhale, press your palms down as you tighten your abdominal muscles and lift your bottom up off the mat.
3. Hold this position for 5 to 10 seconds.
4. Breathe in as you slowly lower your bottom back down to the mat.
5. Repeat 10 times.

Exercise 10: Cat and Camel

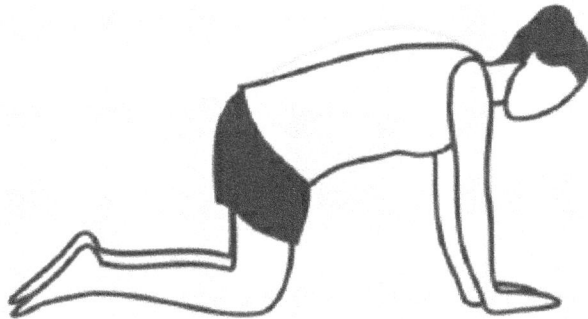

Figure 10: Cat and Camel

The cat-and-camel exercise is helpful for stretching and mobilizing the entire spine.

1. Begin on a yoga mat on your hands and knees.
2. Inhale as you arch your back upward.
3. Exhale as you slowly reverse the bend in your back, bringing your belly down toward the floor.
4. Repeat this movement 10 times in a rhythmic pattern, along with your controlled breathing.

Exercise 11: Side-Stepping with Band

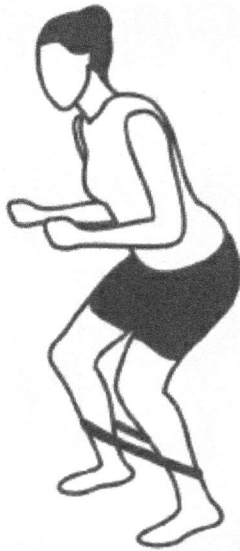

Figure 11: Side Step with Band

Side-stepping with an exercise band is an advanced exercise that strengthens not only the back but also the legs. Choose a resistive therapeutic band, preferably on the lighter or softer side.

1. Wrap the exercise band around your legs below the knees. The band should not be slack when your legs are at shoulder width. The band needs to stay in the same position on your legs throughout the exercise.

2. Slightly bend your knees and place your hands on your hips.

3. With a tight abdomen and buttocks, side-step the length of about 20 feet to one side and return back to the starting point. Keep tension on the therapeutic band throughout the exercise.

4. Repeat 10 times.

Note: Bands can be purchased at Amazon, Walmart, theraband.com, and www.drgracewalkergray.com.

Exercise 12: Monster Walks

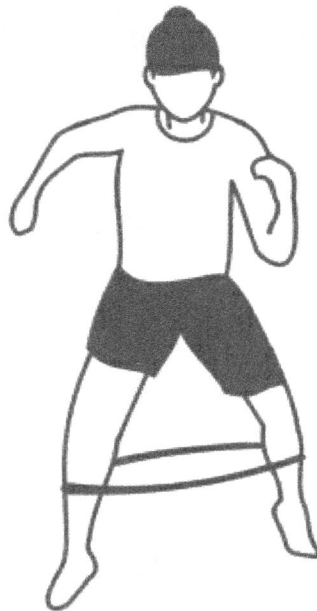

Figure 12: Monster Walk with Band

This exercise is similar to side-stepping with an exercise band, although the movement is forward rather than to the side.

1. Start by wrapping an exercise band around your legs, the same as in the side-stepping exercise.
2. Bend your knees so they are shoulder width apart, hands on your hips.
3. Step forward and away from your body in a semicircular movement. Alternate feet as you step.
4. Keep abdominal and buttocks muscles engaged throughout the movement.
5. Continue the length of about 20 feet and return back to start position.
6. Repeat 10 times.

THREE ACTIVE SIT DISC EXERCISES

During my time completing my postdoctoral fellowship at the Gray Institute, based out of Michigan, I learned about the Fitterfirst Sit Disc (Figure 1). I was so impressed with how it improved my sitting tolerance and my ability to sit and work at a desk that after starting with one, I quickly increased to four: one for each chair I sit in at home and work! In fact, I liked the Sit Disc so much, one Christmas I purchased 150 of them to gift my top referring doctors and close friends. (I did get a great discount for ordering so many!)

I learned how to do three active Sit Disc exercises while I was sitting or working at a computer.

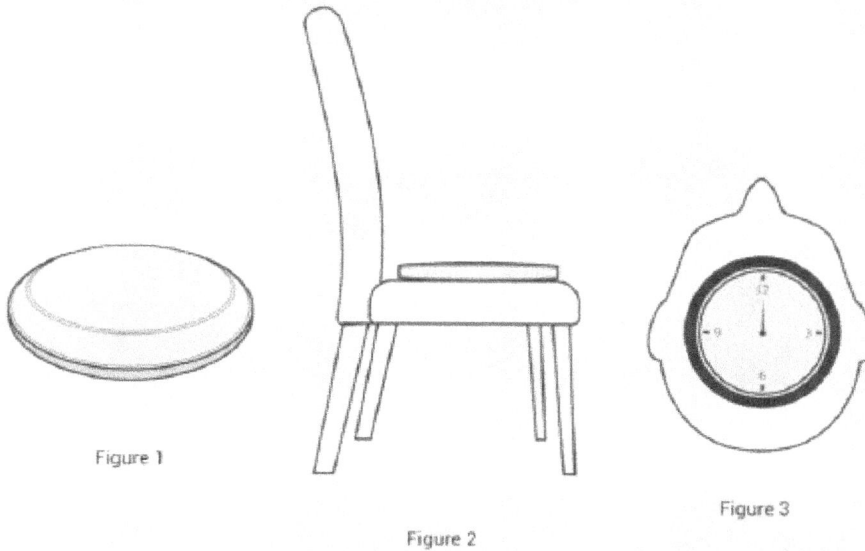

Figure 1

Figure 2

Figure 3

Sit Discs should be placed in the center of a chair (Figure 2). As I seem to be doing a lot on the computer these days, I find myself doing these simple and effective exercises almost hourly.

To understand the concept of exercising on a Sit Disc, imagine a clock sitting on top of your head, with twelve o'clock being in line with your nose (Figure 3). It is important to remember your hips and spine are independent of each other.

Here is the posture set for the three ISO-abs exercises for when you are sitting on the Sit Disc. Place the Sit Disc on a chair. Make sure the chair is an appropriate height: your feet should be flat on the floor and comfortable. Sit tall. Position your shoulders back and down. Now pull your tummy in toward your belly button and hold for the count of five. Repeat ten times.

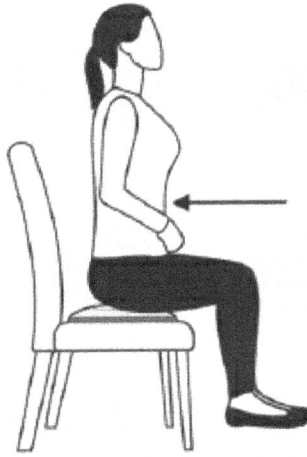

Figure 4

Exercise 1: Rocking Forward and Backward

When you first sit on the Sit Disc, maintain a straight back and keep your shoulders back and down.

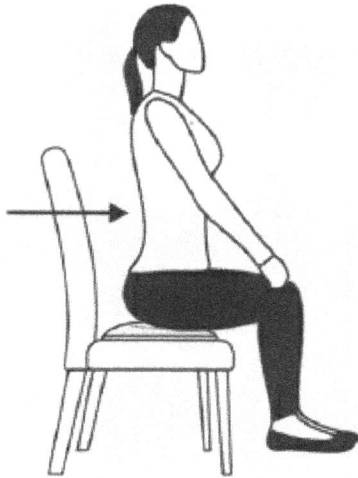

Figure 5

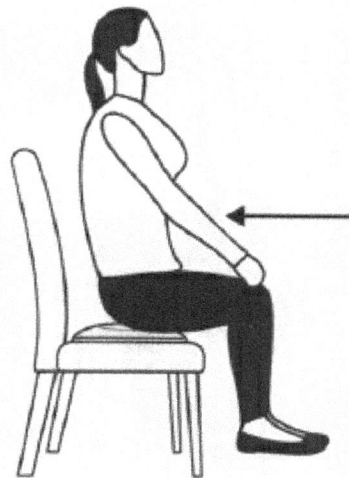

Figure 6

1. Rock forward toward 12 o'clock (Figure 5). Your belly should be sticking out slightly as your back arches.
2. Rock backward toward 6 o'clock (Figure 6). Your belly should be retracted slightly as you flatten your back.
3. Continue rocking back and forth slowly, repeating 10 times.

Exercise 2: Rocking Left and Right

Sit on the Sit Disc with a straight back and your shoulders back and level.

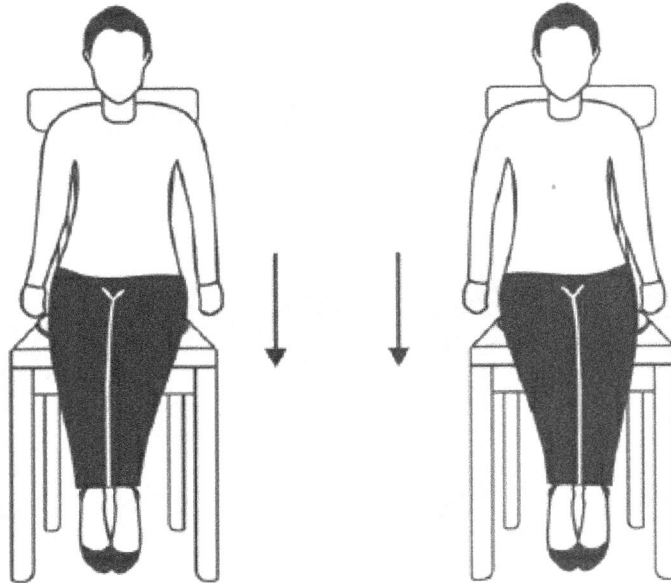

Figure 7   Figure 8

1. Rock to the left side, or 9 o'clock (Figure 7), keeping your shoulders level (no dipping).
2. Rock to the opposite side, or 3 o'clock (Figure 8), keeping shoulders level.
3. Continue rocking left to right slowly, repeating 10 times.

Exercise 3: Rolling Hips Clockwise and Counterclockwise

When you first sit on the disc, sit up straight with your shoulders back.

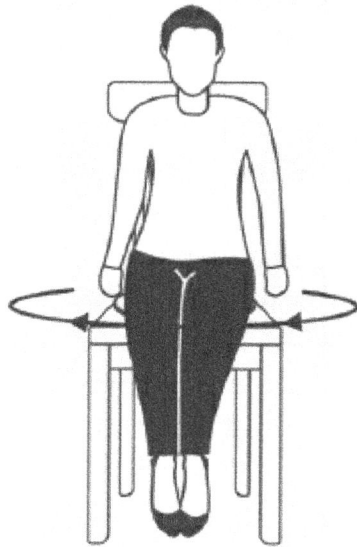 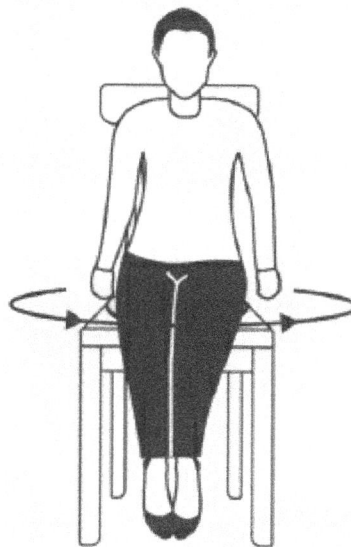

Figure 9   Figure 10

1. Roll your hips clockwise and complete 5 circles in one direction (Figure 9). Go slowly and maintain postural control. Your shoulders should remain level, with no dipping.
2. Roll your hips counterclockwise and complete 5 circles in the opposite direction (Fig. 10).

Sit Discs can be purchased on Amazon. If you happen to weigh over 250 pounds, you may be more comfortable with the large size.

Home exercises may feel uncomfortable, especially if it's been a while since you've attempted to exercise. Fear not—you are not alone. Everyone has to get over the "speed bump" to begin progressing. Unless you notice anything more than soreness, practice while also using ice and joint protection strategies to enable an uninterrupted recovery.

WALKING FOR LOW BACK PAIN

Let's be honest: between sedentary lifestyles at work and home, and poor dietary choices, most of us are not very kind to our lower backs. While it is impossible to change the choices we've made in the past, most of us can adjust our lifestyles moving forward. There is something you can do, something you may already be doing—walking!

A study of over five thousand older adults found that those who walked for exercise were less likely to have low back pain.[11] This was significant because a quarter of the study's participants admitted to experiencing back pain. Another study found that walking at a moderate-to-intense level of effort for twenty to forty minutes, twice a week for six weeks, was as effective as a six-week clinic-based muscle-strengthening program.[12] The Mayo Clinic suggests 150 minutes of moderate aerobic exercise and 75 minutes of vigorous aerobic exercise every week for most healthy adults. Before starting this walking plan, talk with your doctor if you have serious health issues or if you're over forty and you've been inactive recently.

Many people participate in walking for health and exercise. Proper postural techniques and alignment can further reduce strain on your body if you decide to walk for health. Here are two reasons why walking is good for your lower back pain and sciatica.

Walking Keeps You Functional

One of the most frustrating things about low back pain and sciatica is its ability to impact your daily life. It is a difficult realization to discover that even walking has become difficult. However, there are solutions that reduce the strain of walking for exercise, while building strength and endurance.

Walking is important to utilize as exercise because it is an aerobic activity. Aerobic activity is vital to health because it involves increasing your heart rate. An increased heart rate causes blood to flow more quickly, carrying oxygen between your lungs, heart, and muscles. An increase in oxygen throughout the body increases endurance, which allows you to exercise for longer periods of time without getting tired. Ultimately, aerobic exercise helps reduce the risk of developing heart disease.

Think of aerobic exercise as the equivalent of performing an oil change on your car. Dirty oil is flushed out, the oil filter is replaced, and now the engine can run more efficiently with fresh, lubricating oil. Without aerobic exercise, blood can literally pool in the muscles. The muscles need fresh blood and oxygen to perform more efficiently.

Walking also helps to circulate the *synovial fluid* within the joints. Synovial fluid is the thick, stringy fluid within joints that helps lubricate the joint surfaces for ease of movement. Synovial fluid contains hyaluronic acid, lubricin, proteinases, and collagenases. In walking, there is a gentle movement of the lower back's facet joints, which causes this fluid to lubricate all parts of the joint cartilages and aids in healing. Much like blood circulation, synovial fluid lubrication is truly important.

Walking Increases the Production of Endorphins

Endorphins are the body's pain-inhibiting hormones, and walking can encourage their release. Endorphins reduce the amount of perceived pain by binding to the opioid receptors in your brain. If you are able to increase the production of natural endorphins, you may be able to limit your dependence on pain medications. As an added bonus, endorphins help improve your overall mood!

Posture for Walking

Walking can only be an effective exercise if practiced with proper posture. Here are some recommendations for safe walking positions and posture.

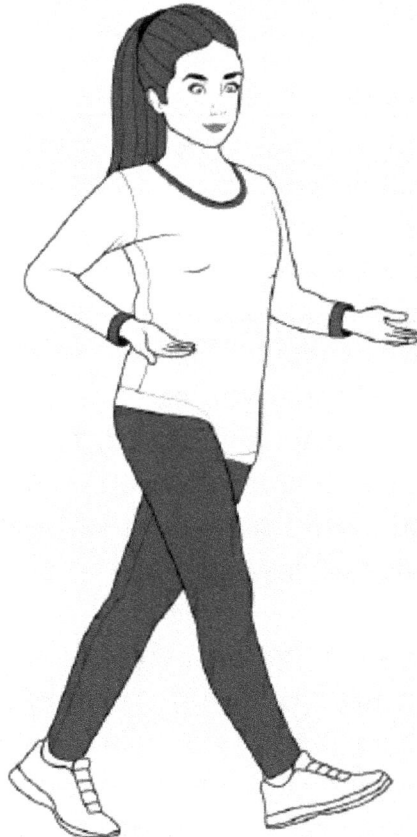

1. Begin walking at a comfortable pace for a few moments with your arms beside your body. Keep your arms close to your body. Keep a straight back, with your shoulders relaxed. Avoid leaning forward or backward, and

keep your chest loose to allow you to breathe well.

2. The arm movement should be in the same direction that you are traveling (forward and backward movements). Do not allow your hands to reach above chin level. While walking, let your elbows swing backward. Your elbows should barely brush the side of your hips with each movement. Keep elbows bent to approximately a right angle, but avoid bending them too much, as this will shorten your stride. Swing your right arm forward as you step forward with your left foot; your left arm swings forward with your right foot. This arm position causes rotation in the thoracic spine, allowing it to absorb some of the shock that walking produces in the lower back.

3. Keep your palms and forearms facing up while you are walking. This will allow you to develop the appropriate rhythm and will keep you from bouncing your arms around, which could be painful for your shoulders and back after a long period.

Starting a Walking Program

Aim to walk for exercise at least five days each week. Start by warming up with a five-minute, slow-paced walk at your leisure. Plan to warm up and cool down for five minutes every time you walk.

Next, speed up to a pace that is comfortable to you. If you are able to walk briskly, try to achieve a speed of around three or four miles an hour. Smartphone applications are available to track your speed. You should be breathing hard, but not so hard that you can't carry on a conversation.

During your first week, attempt to walk for at least five minutes (or as long as you can safely tolerate) after you have completed your warm-up. Next week, add two minutes, for a total of seven minutes of brisk walking each day. Continue adding two minutes of walking each week until you are able to walk a total of thirty minutes.

After you walk, remember to cool down with the same pace of walking that you used during your warm-up. For a more detailed view of what this weekly walking schedule looks like, visit the Mayo Clinic twelve-week walking schedule.

If you have severe back pain or sciatica, it is advisable that you start with a five-minute walk and slowly work your way up to the goal of thirty to forty minutes per day. You can also try walking in a shallow pool. Complete as much walking as you can without instigating pain.

I recently met up with a couple I had treated several years ago. They both said, "Dr. Walker Gray, thank you for helping us. We regularly walk together every morning and have never had another episode of back pain!"

[10] A. Paungmali, L. H. Joseph, P. Sitilertpisan, U. Pirunsan, S. Uthaikhup, "Core stabilization exercise and pain modulation among individuals with chronic nonspecific low back pain," *World Institute of Pain*, November 2017; B. J. Coulombe, "Core stability exercise versus general exercise for chronic low back pain," *Journal of Athletic Training*, January 2017; A. Majeed, A. Ts, A. Sugunan, A. Ms, "The effectiveness of a simplified core stabilization program (TRICCS-Trivandrum Community-based Core Stabilisation) for community-based intervention in chronic non-specific low back pain," *Journal of Orthopaedic Surgery and Research*, March 2019.

[11] Heesang Kim et al, "Association between walking and low back pain in the Korean population: A cross-sectional study," *Annals of Rehabilitation Medicine*, October 2017, doi.org/10.5535/arm.2017.41.5.786.

[12] Ilana Shnayderman, M. Katz-Leurer, "An aerobic walking programme versus muscle strengthening programme for chronic low back pain: A randomized controlled trial," *SAGE Journals*, 31 July 2012, doi.org/10.1177/0269215512453353.

Chapter 6

Solution Three:
Posture and Activities of Daily Living

I am thankful for my studies and learning in becoming a doctor of occupational therapy. I can proudly say that I was the first person in the United States to hold both a doctorate in physical therapy and also a doctorate in occupational therapy. Being trained in both therapies led me to become a well-rounded therapist, and my patients benefitted from this.

This chapter combines both physical therapy and occupational therapy in providing practical solutions for performing everyday activities. In the textbook *Pedretti's Occupational Therapy: Practice Skills for Everyday Functions* (eighth edition), compiled by occupational therapist Mary Pedretti, chapter 41 is an informative section written by Ashley Simon, OTR/L (licensed and registered occupational therapist), on the role of occupational therapy in the treatment of low back pain.[13]

As I read through chapter 41, I realized that Ashley Simon exemplifies exactly what I have taught my clients for decades.

Reducing the pain associated with your low back vertebral column or your sciatic nerve might not be such an expensive endeavor, after all. Making a few adjustments to your everyday habits might be the key. Small changes to how you hold your body up throughout the day could make significant changes to your level of pain. I would like to share the tips that have helped my clients make noticeable changes. Some even found immediate relief.

According to Mary Early, a well-respected occupational therapy researcher, "poor posture is often the underlying culprit in many musculoskeletal diseases."[14] A chronically forward head and slouched posture can contribute to reduced circulation, imbalance of musculature (with the muscles in the chest becoming shortened and the upper back muscles becoming elongated), and fatigue over time.

Having powerful core strength is the foundation of proper body mechanics and posture. Be sure you are following the exercise program described previously to get all the benefits that proper posture can provide you with.

Maintaining healthy posture does require strength. If you find relief from exercise, it is important to remain consistent so you can practice good posture. In all activities of daily living (ADLs), postural control is the key.

STANDING CORRECTLY

Good posture helps keep your bones and joints aligned. This allows your muscles to work more efficiently while minimizing wear on your bones. Poor posture can lead to nerve compression and limited blood flow, which can cause pain and inflammation. Proper posture will help you avoid muscle fatigue, muscle strain, pain, and overuse disorders.

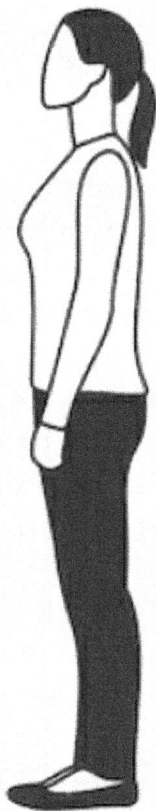

Figure 1: Standing

- Keep your weight over the balls of your feet.
- Slightly bend your knees.

- Spread your feet to shoulder width.
- Keep your arms at the sides of your body, naturally.
- Stand up straight and tall, with your chest out and shoulders back.
- Keep your stomach tight.
- Viewing yourself from the side (in mirrors or with someone else's help), your ears should line up with your shoulder line (there is a tendency to have a forward head).

To maintain a normal standing position for long periods of time, alternate your foot position and make use of a footstool to reduce pressure on your low back. Good posture can reduce the amount of stress on each muscle associated with the back. Achieving good posture is great for preventing back pain.

This is particularly relevant to people who work in jobs where they are required to be on their feet most of the time. In this case, try to obtain a small stool or chair to take the weight off your feet during downtime and to strain your back less.

Posture control is important to keep in mind during functional activities. Over time, many people begin to develop poor posture and balance when standing from a seated position. Many people who develop poor balance over time may attempt to stand without considering where their center of gravity is. It is not uncommon for someone who attempts to stand while leaning too far forward or backward to experience falls.

When standing from a seated position, keep your feet directly under your bottom to use less energy to stand. Be sure to scoot to the edge of the chair before you attempt to stand. Breathe in before you stand and exhale as you stand with a firm belly. This way, your abdominal muscles can assist to support your opposing back muscles.

When available, use upper body support to stand. If you have armrests, or a table or walker in front of you, use them to your advantage. However, do not become overly reliant on using your upper body to do the work your legs are designed to do.

If standing is becoming difficult, do not watch your feet when you stand. It is important to keep your eyes forward if possible. It is not uncommon for someone to experience falls because they shift their gaze from their feet to looking ahead during an attempt to stand.

SITTING CORRECTLY

Sitting for eight hours per day can really cause damage to your back. Examine the chair you use to ensure it has proper support in the lumbar area of your back while both your feet rest flat on the floor (Figure 2a). If you cannot adjust your lumbar support, find a small pillow or rolled-up towel to preserve the arch in your lumbar spine.

As for sitting at a desk, I believe in the rule of 90s—that is, elbows at 90 degrees, hips at 90 degrees, knees at 90 degrees, and ankles at 90 degrees (Figure 2b).

What that looks like is the feet resting flat on the floor or on a footrest, with knees, hips, and elbows all bent at 90 degrees. Your table should be at elbow height, preventing your shoulders from raising up to an uncomfortable position. Be sure that your monitor screen is at an appropriate height. You should be able to look straight ahead at your computer screen. You do not want to feel strained looking up or down at a screen all day.

We can do our best to sit at the desk properly, but understand that there is no *perfect* posture when it comes to sitting at a desk. Our bodies were not designed to sit at desks; such a position is simply not ideal for your body. Be sure you are taking time to get up and stretch. Taking breaks every twenty minutes to get up and move around would be ideal.

If you cannot find a comfortable position sitting at a desk, consider using a standing desk. There are many convertible, or adjustable, desks available that can be used for sitting and standing.

Be careful about sitting on the couch too much, especially if you suffer from sciatica. It has become too easy to "binge watch" TV all day on the couch. Please be sure to get up at least once every hour for at least five minutes. Take this time to walk the dog or grab the mail.

Lastly, your driving position is an important issue. Driving can be difficult on the body. The factors that can cause injuries just driving a car every day include applying constant pressure on the wheel and pedals, hunching over the center console, wedging your knee into the steering column, and receiving the vibrations from the steering wheel.

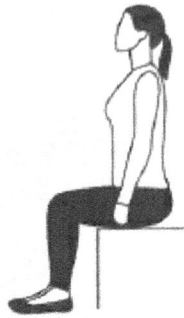

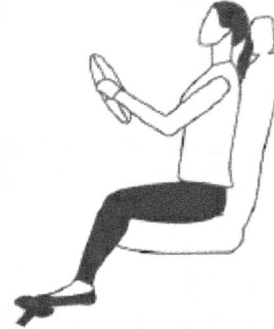

Figure 2a: Sitting at Desk   Figure 2b: Sitting at a Computer   Figure 2c: Sitting in Car

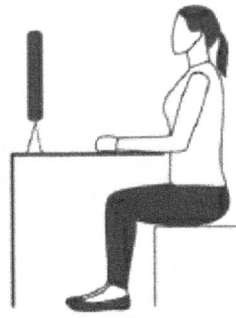

Cars today are designed with ergonomics in mind. Whether we choose to utilize these features is up to us. Similar to how we sit at a desk, the rule of 90 is again important. If you feel increased pressure in your hips or lower back, try adjusting the seat up or down next time you come to a safe stop (Figure 2c). Also, make sure the car seat is close enough to the steering wheel for your comfort. Sometimes the seat may be too far away from the dash, causing your legs to stretch out abnormally, which results in irregular forces on the low back. This might occur when two separate drivers share the same car. Be sure you are getting out and walking around during long trips, too. A break once an hour for five minutes is recommended.

PUSHING AND PULLING

Posture when pushing or pulling objects is an afterthought for most. However, pushing and pulling motions can be very dangerous. Many people experience lower back pain or sciatica from attempting to twist while pushing or pulling.

To push, pull your tummy in, bend your legs in a walking stance, keep your elbows close to your sides, and push as you breathe out (Figure 3a). To pull, pull your tummy in, bend your legs in a walking stance, keep your elbows close to your sides, and pull as you breathe out (Figure 3b). While our bodies can push and pull very large items, it is very important to avoid twisting motions while moving objects. That is a surefire way to cause back pain.

If you find you need to move an object, be sure you are bending your knees rather than your back.

Of course, if you can find help to move an object, find it! Heavy objects can wait for help!

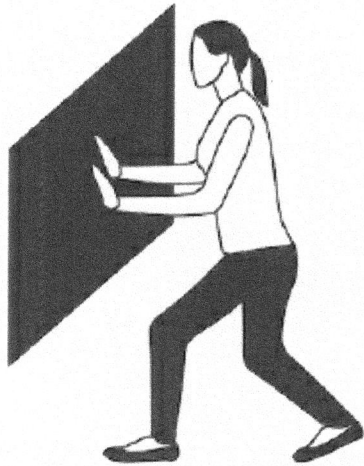

Figure 3a: Pushing

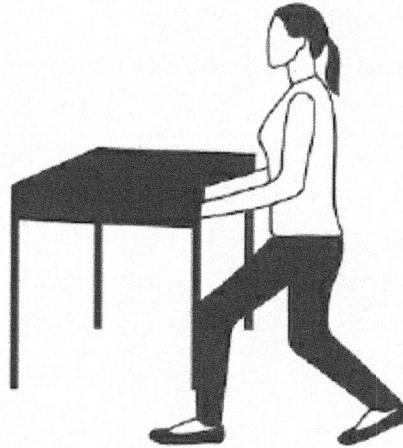

Figure 3b: Pulling

CHOOSING A MATTRESS

Research shows that people who sleep on beds that fill the contour of their spine are less likely to suffer from back pain.[15] Pillows shouldn't be too high, and there shouldn't be any gaps between the body and the mattress.

Beds are a big investment, but if we break down how much your old mattress is costing you in pain, lack of energy, and work efficiency, you might consider selling your car to go get a new mattress right now!

Picking a good mattress can be difficult. Everyone has a differently shaped body and has different preferences. Find a mattress that fills the contour of your back and supports your entire body evenly. Many mattress stores have warranties and buy-back guarantees, which might be a good resource to pay for once your mattress has settled down and broken in. I usually find that a mattress is good for ten years and at that point you should consider replacing it.

Interestingly enough, at a recent social function I met a patient I had treated years ago. She said, "Dr. Walker Gray, you recommended that I get a new mattress for my bed. So, I did! And that was the key! My back pain went away! Thank you for the advice!"

Sleeping positions are nearly as important as sitting positions at a desk. You spend (hopefully) between five and nine hours in bed each night; proper alignment is critical during sleep.

Pillows should be positioned to allow your head to flow with the natural curvature of your spine. Those of us who choose to sleep on our backs (Figure 4a) should consider placing a pillow under our knees. A pillow under the knees brings the spine to a natural, neutral position. Of course, a proper pillow under the head is important as well. Some find the most comfort with two pillows under their head—one to raise their shoulders and another to raise their head slightly above their shoulders.

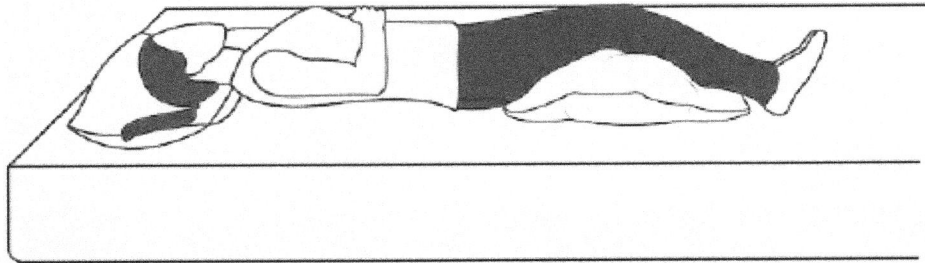

Figure 4a: Sleeping on Back

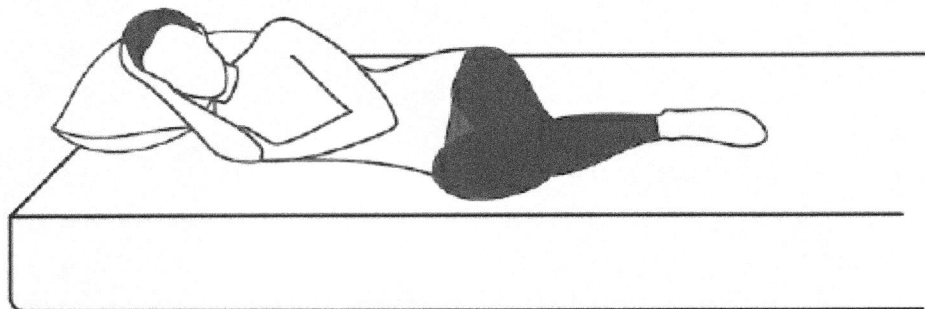

Figure 4b: Sleeping on Side

Side sleepers (Figure 4b) may find the most comfort with a pillow between their knees. A pillow between the knees relieves pressure from the hips and keeps the lumbar (lower) spine straight. A pillow under your head will keep your neck alignment straight. Be sure it's not too thick or thin. Lastly, be sure you are not putting too much pressure through your shoulder. The shoulder making contact with the bed should be slightly forward (protraction).

Inadequate sleep can lead to dysregulation in the body and increased pain. During bouts of pain, sleep can be difficult. Unfortunately, this could lead to a vicious cycle of pain and lack of sleep in people who experience lower back pain or sciatica. You need to have good sleep in order to heal!

It is important to be informed about the dangers of lack of sleep. Stimulating activities—such as using the phone or watching TV—should be avoided for at least an hour prior to sleep. In occupational therapy this practice is called *sleep hygiene*.

Sleep hygiene isn't limited to electronics use. Activities such as house cleaning or laundry should also be avoided at least an hour before sleep. To properly calm down for sleep, it is important to "ramp down" your activity level in order to fall asleep swiftly. As you prepare for bed, complete your activities from most stimulating to least stimulating. For example, complete household cleaning chores, spend some time watching television, enter the bedroom to read a book, and then consider some light stretching or aromatherapy before finally attempting sleep. Maybe you can imagine why it would be difficult to fall asleep if those tasks were done in reverse order!

Activities that would be appropriate just before sleep include warm showers, calming music, aromatherapy, herbs and CBD oil, relaxing stretching, and massage, which we will discuss in detail later in this book. Try focusing on the breathing techniques and body-consciousness techniques mentioned later in this book while falling asleep. Sleep hygiene plans can be individualized to your liking. Experiment to find which routine suits you best.

GETTING OUT OF BED

How many people do you know who severely hurt their backs by simply getting out of bed? It is quite common. Be conscious about how you wake up and get out of bed. You can "log roll" to the edge of the bed.

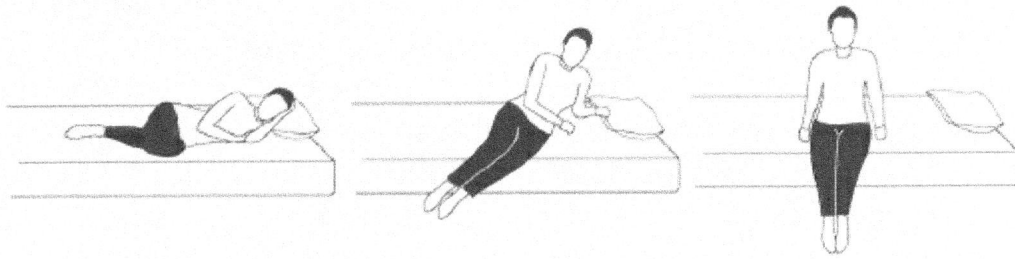

Figure 3: Getting up Out of Bed

- Lying on your side, use your arms to help push you to the end of the bed.
- Allow your feet to hang off the edge of the bed for a while before you attempt to sit up; this way gravity can assist you.
- It is important to have your bed at an appropriate height to stand. You should not have a bed that is too low. A bed that is too low can be extremely difficult to stand from. Conversely, a bed that is too high can be difficult to get into. If need be, a walker at your bedside can be helpful for upper-body support when standing from the bed.
- Most importantly, take your time getting up from bed. Perform a self-assessment and get up slowly rather than springing to your feet. Getting up slowly allows your blood pressure to normalize after sleeping.
- Finally, when you sit up from the bed, be conscious of your back. After you have been stationary and resting for so long, you are extremely vulnerable to straining your body. Be sure to practice using your arms where you can, to help with activities like getting out of bed or standing from the car.

DRESSING

Dressing can be surprisingly difficult for someone who suffers from sciatica or low back pain. Tasks such as pulling up pants or reaching down to pull on socks and tie shoes can be very painful. There are a variety of adaptive pieces of equipment and some techniques to reduce pain during dressing.

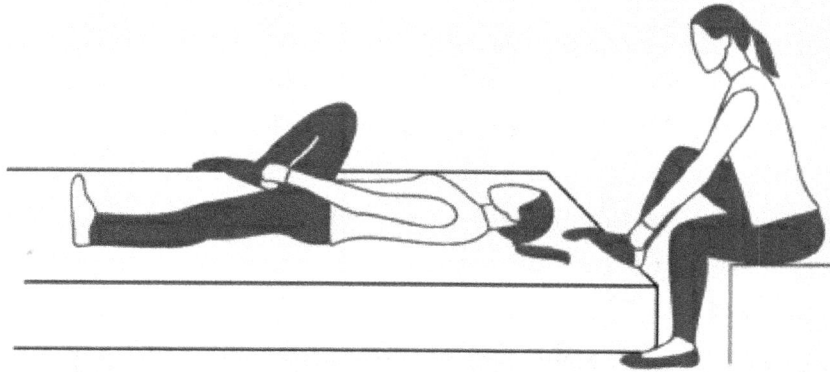

Figure 6: Dressing

Shoes and Socks

Shoes and socks can be some of the most difficult clothing items to manage for those experiencing pain as a result of sciatica or low back pain. One helpful method for putting on your socks or shoes from a seated position is to bring one leg up and cross that ankle over the opposite resting knee. If you have had a hip replacement, consult your doctor before attempting this movement; it could be against your doctor's recommendation.

Fortunately, many assistive devices are used by physical and occupational therapists to simplify these tasks. Here is a list:

- Sock aids to apply socks without bending your back
- Long-arm shoehorns to help you slide your feet into your shoes without bending down
- Well-fitting slip-on shoes to reduce shoelace tying
- A long-arm reacher to help grab shoes or socks from the floor to avoid bending down

Lower-Body Dressing

Lower-body dressing is another task that can be difficult for someone experiencing pain, especially if their strength or balance is not as good as it used to be. Lower-body dressing is important, because putting on a pair of pants or undergarments can be very dangerous. Think about it: when you're placing your legs into leg holes, looking down or maybe hunched over, you are at a high risk of falling.

Here are some suggestions to reduce strain and increase safety while dressing your lower body:

- Practice putting your pants on from a seated position. Put both legs in the holes while seated on a stable surface. Once you have slid your pants up to your knees, you can stand with more stability on both feet to pull your pants up to your hips. Use a walker or stable surface to help yourself to a standing position with arm and hand support if need be.
- Use a long-arm reacher to help you grab your pants. Pant legs can be bunched up and grabbed with the reacher arm to help guide your feet inside the holes.
- Use a walker or other solid surface for arm and hand support while pulling your pants up.
- If you choose to dress your lower body while standing, consider propping your back against a strong wall.
- If standing or sitting is painful, you can put your pants on in bed, too. Lying on your back and bending your knees can help you put your pants on, one leg at a time.

Upper-Body Dressing

While upper-body dressing is not usually affected by back pain or sciatica, there are some things to keep in mind to reduce any strain or pain that may occur while you are dressing your upper body. Dressing your upper body can also be dangerous. Your eyes might be covered and your arms may get tangled inside your shirt.

Consider the following tips:

- If you are having a difficult time dressing your lower body, consider sitting while you perform upper-body dressing. You may want to save all of your energy to dress your lower body.
- Sitting is the safest way to dress your upper body. If your arms are tied up in your shirt and you can't see, any loss of balance can make for a dangerous situation!
- Using a long-arm reacher can be helpful to reach for clothes stored up high or down low.
- If back pain makes it difficult to put on and take off a T-shirt, consider wearing button-up shirts. Dressing sticks are available to help you get your arms in the holes.

WALKING THE DOG

Walking the dog is a necessary task for many people. Many people have poor body mechanics during this task—keeping their head or shoulders slouched forward, or holding the leash improperly.

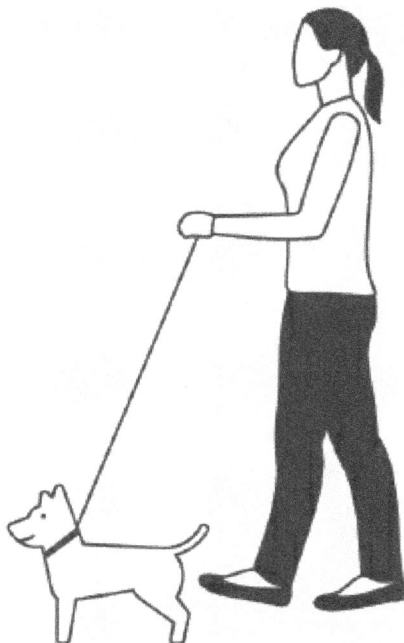

Figure 7: Walk the Dog

- When walking the dog, remember to keep your head and shoulders aligned over your trunk. Your arms should be bent in a 90-degree angle and kept close to your core.
- Holding the leash with two hands can be very helpful in case Fido decides to go after that squirrel or cat. Keep both hands close to your abdomen, near the belly button. Many accidents and injuries happen while walking the dog, and they happen fast! Be ready and maintain good posture.

CARING FOR YOUR PET

No matter if you have a pet mouse or a Saint Bernard, pet care must be done with good ergonomics and positioning. Use good body mechanics, with a neutral spine, when squatting or kneeling to pet or groom your pet.

- Long-handled scoopers for picking up pet waste are available to reduce strain on your back.
- Self-dispensing water bowls are available to reduce the amount of bending you do. Or consider pouring water from a standing position, if you are able

to do so without making a mess.

- People with larger dogs should avoid jerking and twisting motions when playing with their dog.

DOING THE LAUNDRY

Laundry is another overlooked task. Laundry involves heavy lifting and some awkward motions. Be sure to make multiple trips to carry laundry—do not try to carry it all in one load. (You probably dropped a sock in the hallway, anyhow. Remember to bend your knees to pick it up.)

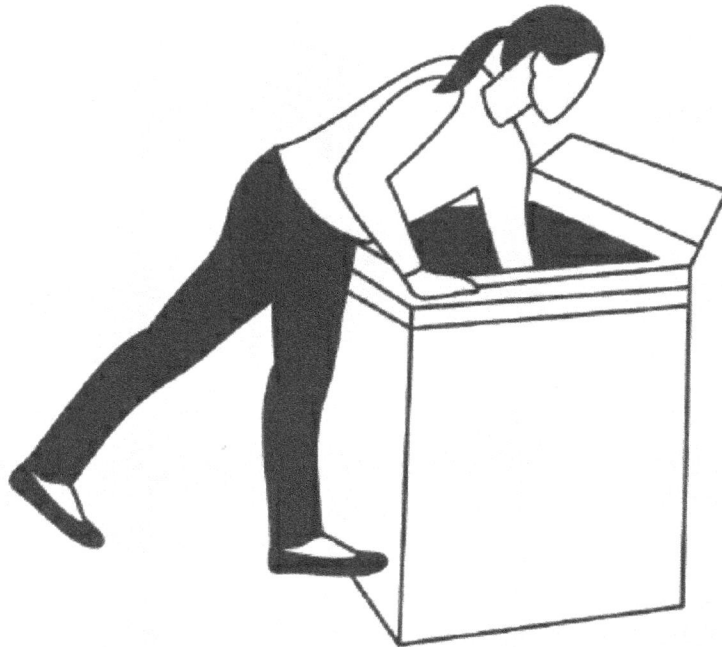

Figure 8: Laundry

- For front-load washer-dryer units, squat down with your knees rather than your back. If you find you have to squat in the laundry room often, consider leaving a folding chair tucked in the laundry room to help.
- For top-loading units, avoid hunching over the appliance. You should avoid trying to carry items from a washer to a dryer in a forward position because you will be twisting while carrying a load (a big no-no).
- Anti-slip mats with some padding in front of your washer-dryer unit can be

helpful additions to reduce pressure in your legs and spine, as well as increase safety.

- Raised laundry platforms are available to increase the height of laundry appliances. Raising the height of laundry units allows for easier access and reduced strain while performing laundry tasks. Raised laundry platforms can be found on Amazon and at local appliance stores.

TOILETING

Toileting is an often-overlooked task. The bathroom can be an extremely dangerous place, considering the sharp edges on tubs and sinks, as well as glass and mirrors.

- When attempting to sit or stand from the toilet, practice proper body mechanics. Be sure to keep your center of gravity upon sitting and standing, by keeping your feet under your bottom as much as possible. Use your knees to squat down rather than bending your back.

- If you find you are having a difficult time, consider upper-body support to sit and stand. A walker in the bathroom can be a very good investment, even if it's only used to sit and stand from the toilet. Other options, such as over-the-toilet commodes and grab-bar installations, can be very wise investments as well.

ENJOYING SEXUAL ACTIVITY

Sexual activity can be enjoyed in safe positions. It is important to remember to keep a neutral spine whenever possible (Figures 9a and 9b). If you experience pain during back extension (bending backward), a rolled towel under your upper back or bottom during activity can help keep you in a neutral position. If spinal flexion (forward) is painful, a rolled towel under your lower back may help keep you in a safe position.

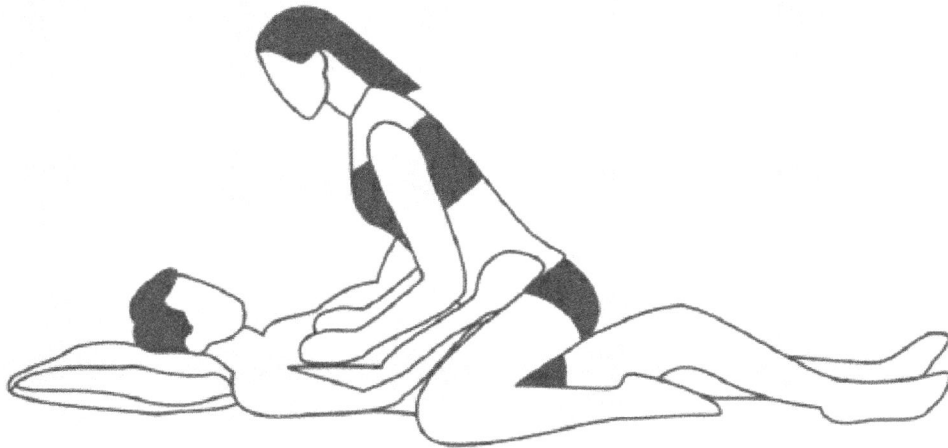

Figure 9a: Sexual Activity

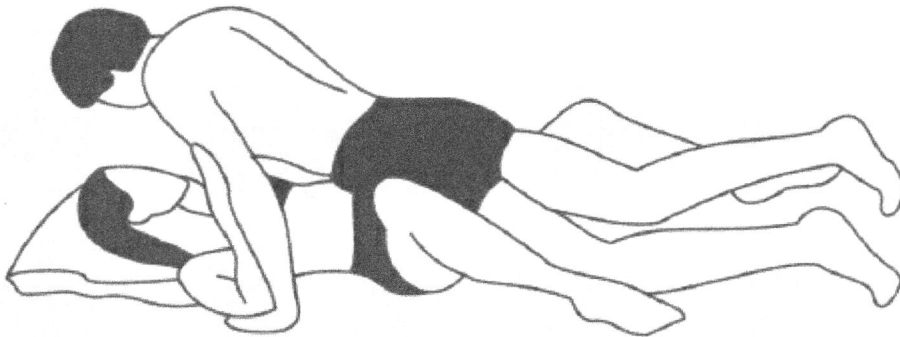

Figure 9b: Sexual Activity

- Some men and women find a foam wedge under the legs or behind the back can be helpful to find a comfortable position.
- In addition, for men, standing and placing one foot in front of the other will encourage good alignment.

CLEANING THE HOUSE

It can be very difficult to clean without hunching your back. There are some helpful tools to reduce the strain cleaning can put on your body.

- Consider bringing with you a foam pad as a kneeler when you are working on your knees.
- Avoid bending and twisting motions, especially while carry a load.
- Use long-arm tools, such as toilet brushes and dusters.

DOING YARDWORK

This is another task that could benefit from using a foam pad under the knees as a kneeler, especially during pruning and planting tasks.

- If you are doing work that can be completed on a raised surface to allow for better body mechanics, do so. This is a great way to prevent incorrect posture for extended periods of time.
- Use caution when using machinery or handheld tools that require bad posture for use. Tools such as weed whackers and leaf blowers can put a tremendous strain on the body because of their weight. Many tools used for yardwork require you to carry objects and twist. Avoid twisting with a heavy load; instead turn with your feet and lower with your legs.

MANAGING THE HOME

This might sound simple, but it is rare for many people to follow this rule: Keep your most often-used items in accessible places! You should not be picking up and storing heavy items down low! Organization is key.

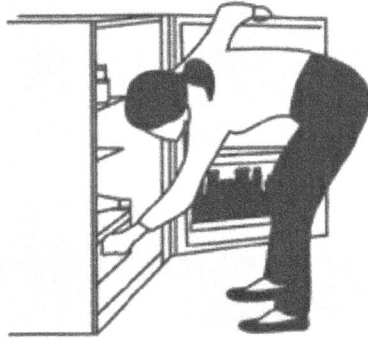

Figure 10a: Home Organization: Refrigrator

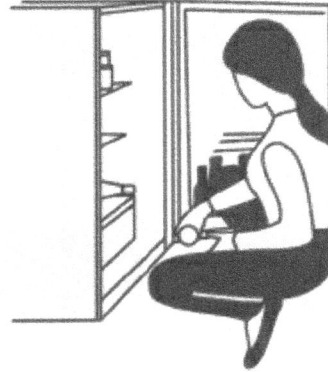

Figure 10b: Home Organization: Refrigrator

- In your refrigerator, place heavy items around abdominal height. You do not want to have to lift a gallon of milk from the bottom shelf if you don't have to.
- The same principle applies to the pantry and dishes.
- Figure 10a shows a picture of a woman using her back to bend, **which is incorrect**.
- Figure 10b shows a woman using her knees to bend down, allowing her spine to remain straight. **This is the correct way** to bend down for items.

LIFTING

Much as it is with pushing and pulling, it is important to avoid twisting motions while lifting and carrying objects. Use the strong leg muscles in your thighs to squat rather than straining your back muscles to lift items.

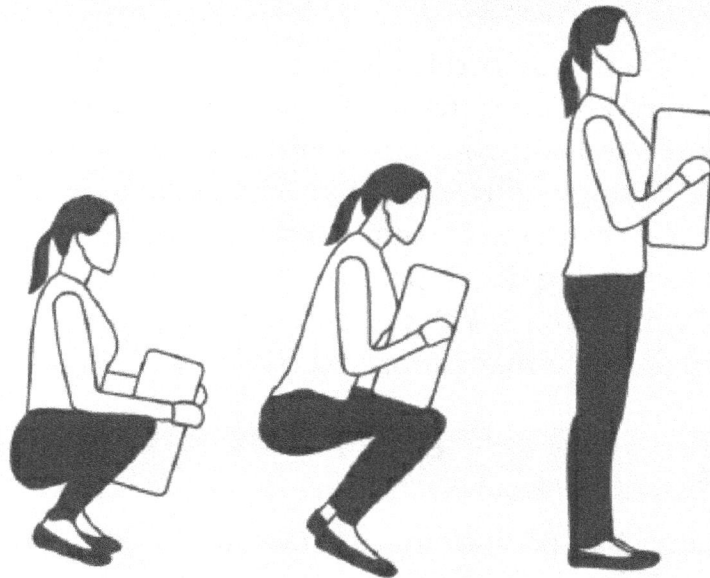

Figure 10c: Lifting

- Bend down to the right level with your knees. Avoid raising or twisting with your back; take the extra few steps to turn your entire body instead. Learning to use the correct methods will put less strain on your back.
- Remember to keep a firm belly and engage your abdominal core muscles. This way, your abdominal muscles can help support your opposing back muscles. And remember to breathe out as you lift.
- Be sure to plan your movements ahead of time, to allow yourself to use your strong leg muscles rather than your back.
- If something is too heavy to lift, get help from a friend or neighbor. If you can find a dolly or cart to use for help, use it!

People who lift with their back suffer from injuries much more easily. Here is what Valerie A. wrote to me, "I spent twenty years working for the US Postal Service and never thought I would experience back pain, since I was always moving. One day it hit me, and I found myself sitting on the sidewalk halfway through my route. I'd made an awkward motion trying to carry a heavy package and my back completely gave out.

"I went to meet Dr. Grace Walker Gray, and learned that I had been carrying and lifting the wrong ways for twenty years. A quick correction in my technique, and a lot of ice, and I was back on the road!"

Enjoying Leisure Time

Some leisure activities encourage bad body mechanics. From cycling to fishing to knitting, it is always important to remember to keep a neutral body position. Keep your shoulders relaxed and your knees and elbows at 90 degrees if your leisure activity allows. Lifting and twisting should be avoided if possible.

If your leisure activity causes you pain, consider reassessing your activity. New products are always being developed to allow people to do the things they love with proper body mechanics. Your research can pay off and allow you to enjoy your leisure activities for many more years!

Traveling

It can be easy to fall into bad positioning and posture on long car rides or in airplanes. The result is pain, stiffness, and even more muscle cramps. The problems can be exacerbated if you sit in a twisted position, lean off to one side, or fall asleep with your neck and head out of alignment.

- First, and most important, align your spine! A small pillow or towel in the small of your back could make all the difference. If you plan on flying, a neck pillow could be a wise investment.
- If you are on a plane with headrests, keep the back of your head in the center of the headrest. Some plane headrests bend on each side to cradle your head in a supportive position. Take advantage of that feature.
- If you decide to read, be sure to bring your book or tablet up toward your head to prevent straining your neck and back to look down.
- Be sure to shift your body occasionally to avoid pressure points.
- Maintain 90-degree bends at your hips, knees, elbows, and ankles by repositioning your seat and armrests if possible.
- If you ride on a plane or in a train, be sure to get up and stretch when you can.

It can be difficult to obtain proper positioning when you travel— especially on an airplane. If you are prepared with any pillows or assistive devices that will make your trip more comfortable, you are ahead of the game. Take time before you travel next and try some techniques or products that may alleviate or reduce your pain. Don't hesitate to purchase a neck pillow or a phone or tablet stand to reduce neck strain. Many companies will take your returns if you find out their product is not helpful.

CONSERVING ENERGY

The general principle of energy conservation is about working smarter rather than harder. Energy conservation requires us to plan ahead, set priorities, monitor activity tolerance, eliminate unnecessary tasks, and save energy.

Energy conservation techniques are numerous. It is important to recognize areas where you can conserve energy in your own life. A few energy conservation techniques that you could employ when getting ready for a lunch party might include these methods:

- Plan ahead: Shop one to two days prior to the event. Chop and prepare food one day ahead of the party.
- Prioritize: Do not attempt other events at the same time. Focus on the most immediate or important one at hand.
- Eliminate unnecessary tasks: Go out to eat breakfast and dinner to save energy for making lunch.
- Share responsibilities: Make the main course and have others bring side plates.
- Decrease energy required for a task: Sit while you prepare food rather than stand. Keep your most-used utensils close by.

Energy conservation is simple, but it can be very difficult to practice day to day. Be sure to plan a day or two ahead of strenuous activity and give yourself time to consider energy conservation techniques.

PACING YOUR ACTIVITY

Activity pacing is the act of monitoring your energy level between periods of work and rest. It may sound simple, but it can be difficult to keep track of your energy when work needs to get done.

For example, consider our lunch party scenario. During the various activities for getting ready, it is important to monitor how you are feeling. Give yourself enough time to take rest breaks if you begin to fatigue or experience pain.

The bigger picture of activity pacing is knowing your body well enough to know when it is time to take a break or save the work for another day. Constantly pushing your body to its limit is not healthy. Bodies require rest!

Personally, I practice what I preach. My work station is ergonomically set up, and I have several travel aides that make flying easier. My kitchen is organized and I monitor how I lift and bend. Most importantly, I ask my husband for help if I need it. When I go out for lunch or dinner with my friends, they frequently comment on my erect posture at the table.

[13] Ashley Simon, "Chapter 41," in: Lorraine Williams Pedretti, ed., *Pedretti's Occupational Therapy: Practice Skills for Physical Dysfunction*, 8th ed., St. Louis: Elsevier, 2018.

[14] Mary Early, *Physical Dysfunction Practice Skills for the Occupational Therapy Assistant*, St. Louis: Elsevier, 2006.

[15] *Mayo Clinic*, "Slide show: Sleeping positions that reduce back pain," 21 May 2014, www.mayoclinic.org/diseases-conditions/back-pain/multimedia/sleeping-positions/sls-20076452?s=3.

Chapter 7

Solution Four:
Professional Treatments

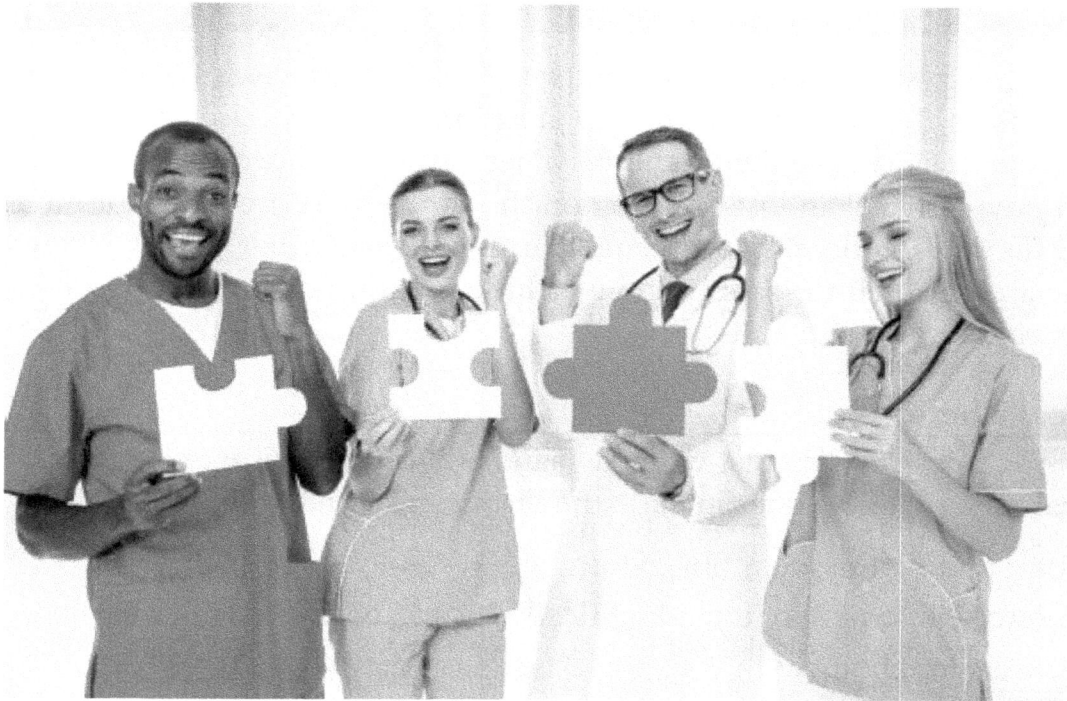

Once age catches up with us, each ache and pain begins to direct our way of life. Even sitting at the computer or driving becomes a daunting task, let alone participating in our favorite physical activity. We all experience pain differently. Some prefer to rest until the pain subsides. Others opt for the pain relief provided by massage.

Massage is the quickest way to relieve pain in the neck, the back, and other parts of the body. People forget about this little relief too often. Some prefer to bandage the problem with pills from their doctor. While medication does work for pain relief, it does not solve the underlying issue.

ARE THERE ANY SPECIALISTS OUT THERE?

Visiting a specialist is the best option for low back pain and sciatica. There are many health professionals who treat these conditions and each may have a different approach. These include family doctors, physical therapists, occupational therapists, chiropractors and massage therapists. If pain is severe, or showing any of the "red flags' reported in Part I Chapter 3 then this may indicate going to a spine specialist.

PHYSICAL THERAPISTS, OCCUPATIONAL THERAPISTS, AND CHIROPRACTORS

Physical therapists, occupational therapists, and chiropractors focus on the solution using therapies that deal with joint functions, exercise, and movement. These practices do have their benefits. They can show more attention to the entire body, rather than just focusing on the problem. A great deal of time is wasted finding solutions to problems that don't exist, rather than working on a specific area. Sometimes, applying just a little pressure to a muscle knot might be the answer.

Physical Therapists

Look for a physical therapist who has hands-on mobilization experience. Physical therapy techniques include the following:

- Joint and soft tissue mobilization
- Exercise instruction, including flexibility and core strengthening
- Self-care techniques
- Postural and ergonomic advice
- Ice pack and cryotherapy (cold therapy)
- Trigger point therapy
- ML830 laser treatments (See chapter 10)
- Kinesiology taping

Occupational Therapists

Occupational therapists perform evaluations to assess a patient's abilities to perform activities of daily living (ADLs) and to help patients understand back protection techniques and pain behaviors. Therapists guide patients to manage their low back and sciatic pain by teaching them problem-solving skills and identifying realistic lifestyle changes. Patients are educated in proper body mechanics, anatomy, work simplification, relaxation, and adaptive techniques to help with ADL performance.[16] Many occupational therapists are also trained to teach mindfulness meditation techniques.

Massage Therapists

Massage therapists have the most hands-on experience of all therapists regarding treating muscles, but they seem to know very little about myofascial pain syndrome. Furthermore, their training standards are inconsistent. However, I have run across several excellent massage therapists who work effectively with trigger points. It's worthwhile asking your doctor or friends for recommendations.

A former client, Dave, said, "Physical therapy was going very well, but my progress began to plateau. I was looking for something else to help get me through the soreness that can come with exercise. I found that a weekly visit to a recommended massage therapist really made a difference."

Self-massage techniques provide the same benefits as directed massages. While seeing a good massage therapist can be an expense, remember that your pain relief is a priority. There's nothing like a good massage to help relieve pain. Work and exercise can be hard, especially as we age. We become sore more easily. We end up in odd positions to try to ease the pain. Perhaps you have decided to opt out of exercise because the soreness was too intense last time.

As difficult as it may be, we must not discredit exercise. Exercise is an important tool to heal and preserve health. One must remember that with increased exercise, increased soreness may be a result. When we exercise, muscle fibers are literally ripping and tearing apart, and then they heal. This process is natural; increased muscle strength is a result. The process is exhausting and sometimes painful. You must have a way to combat this to continue exercising and preserving your health. This is what makes massage so essential as part of the healing process.

When you begin a new exercise regimen, you can expect to get sore. Perhaps you are experiencing *knots*. These pains and aches are caused by trigger points, which are malfunctioning knots of muscle tissue. See "Strange Aches and Trigger Points" below for more information regarding knots and trigger points.

I treat myself to at least one massage per month. I may get my massage from an experienced and licensed massage therapist, or I may get it from a physical therapist who is also a licensed massage therapist. I have a wonderful chiropractor whom I see twice a month. I regularly use tennis balls in self-massage treatments. And I may have a need for physical therapy every two years or so. If so, then I will ask for kinesiology taping if needed. Finally, I follow occupational therapy ADL advice, as it is ingrained in me after all my training.

Chiropractors

For some, there is nothing more satisfying than a trip to the chiropractor. For others, there is nothing more terrifying. The sounds of joints cracking and popping can be intimidating, especially when you are in pain. However, it is important to know that chiropractic therapy is not as simple as that.

Chiropractic therapy involves the manipulation of the musculoskeletal system. Practitioners adjust joints, typically including the spine. Chiropractic therapy is focused on treating the ailments related to the nervous system.

Although it is described as a noninvasive, alternative form of medicine, chiropractic adjustments give most people tremendous relief. Chiropractors with the most hands-on experience have a great deal of competency with a variety of patients. A good chiropractor can help provide pain relief with little trial and error.

Chiropractic techniques include the following:

- Full-body manipulation
- Self-care techniques
- Postural and ergonomic advice
- Nutritional recommendations
- Ice pack and cryotherapy

STRANGE ACHES AND TRIGGER POINTS

Referred pain, also known as reflective pain, is pain that is perceived at a location other than the site of the painful stimulus. Trigger points are interesting because of their ability to cause pain in unrelated areas. Many clients with carpal tunnel syndrome or epicondylitis (an inflammatory condition of condyles also known as tennis elbow) have had enormous relief from trigger point therapy.

Sciatica and Other Nerve Problems

Many people believe that sciatica stems from trigger point irritation. This is not true. Sciatica is caused by inflammation or irritation to the sciatic nerve, which exits from the lumbar (lower) spine and runs down the back of the leg.

What Is a Trigger Point?

There are many trigger points that are often mistaken for nerve problems. Fortunately, a nerve test administered by a physician can determine whether or not a problem is associated with a nerve.

Myofascial pain syndrome affects the tissue that covers the muscle, called the *fascia*. It can affect one muscle or a group of muscles. If you are experiencing increased pain from these trigger points, you may want to ask your physician about myofascial pain syndrome.

These sensitive areas of muscle groups are often irritated by being overworked or from an injury. Knots are not muscle fibers that are tangled, they just feel that way. Trigger points often lead to having small tightened muscles, which can be extremely painful.

While there is no definitive research, it is believed that small areas of muscles can cut off their own blood supply, which can lead to pain in the immediate area. Myofascial trigger points can be incredibly painful and difficult to diagnose.

A myofascial trigger point is an irritated area in the fascia, or connecting tissue, within the skeletal muscle fiber. They begin as tender nodules that contain taut bands of muscle fibers that have contracted and failed to relax. This is where the term *knots* comes from. The term *trigger point* came about in 1942 by Janet Travell, MD, after a patient reacted in pain from being touched in the affected area. Trigger points can occur simultaneously throughout the body. They can occur anywhere. Trigger points are delicate areas of the body that can cause discomfort in other regions of the body. Often, they are sensitive areas in a muscle causing pain.

There are many thoughts regarding the mysterious aches and pains that we feel are related to trigger points. Many people are not aware of the body's ability to expel wasteful toxins. Many back pain issues are linked to toxins that form knots that cause pain.

The characteristics of the myofascial trigger point include these symptoms:

- The painful area of muscle is not caused by an external injury, inflammation, trauma, degradation, or infection.
- The affected area is characterized by a nodule that, once stimulated, results in the muscle in the area twitching.
- The trigger point may palpitate (push into) and continue to radiate pain in the area and sometimes elsewhere.

Trigger points are thought to be the leading causes of muscle aches and pains. These aches and pains can be in the form of headaches, neck pain, and lower back pain.

Trigger points are usually the cause for various discomforts:

- Constant pain issues: Trigger points are natural and everyone has them, but at some point, they are going to cause pain.

- Other pain issues: Trigger points can be confusing; count on them to show up after an injury or painful muscular issue.
- Pain issues that mimic other pains: Trigger points can mimic toothaches and headaches. They can be easily misdiagnosed.

Let's Take a Closer Look at Trigger Points

Trigger point therapy is not overly complicated, but it is not an exact science, either. Many agree that muscle pain is an important subject, while trigger points still appear to be a work in progress.

Here are some topics to consider:

- Accurate theories regarding trigger points
- What's true and what is false
- Who disagrees and why

There are some theories that seem odd but are backed by good research. There are other theories that may have come from outer space. Trigger point research is often overlooked in favor of other more critical areas that demand more research. Musculoskeletal medicine has made great strides recently and is getting some real attention. Chronic pain is so common today; everyone has different reasons how or why they are in pain. Doctors are flooded by the topic, though in many cases they don't bother to understand it.

Trigger points are likely a dysfunction within the muscle tissue, but that theory is still unproven. Therefore, the topic remains on hold, with no signs of being picked up. Skeletal muscle is the largest organ in the body.[17] It is complex and vulnerable to injury and dysfunction. Dysfunction is typically caused by simple wear and tear from daily activities. A doctor's attention often turns to the bones, joints, nerves and bursae, rather than the trigger points.

Trigger points are difficult to diagnose due to their internal nature. The phenomenon is nearly in the alternative-medicine realm and is often misdiagnosed by conventional medical doctors.

Severe Symptoms

There have been cases of trigger points causing severe symptoms that have led to mistaken medical emergencies. In one case a man was rushed to the hospital with severe arm pain and was treated for a heart attack. After a series of tests, his doctor was able to relieve his pain by simply stimulating his pectoral muscle to relax the trigger point.

Who Understands and Treats Trigger Points?

Therapy for trigger points is still evolving. Many of the best therapists are the ones with the most hands-on experience treating trigger points. It is important to understand: there is no one way to treat trigger point pain. Techniques that involve stimulating the trigger point have better results with some people, and other techniques work better with others. It is a process, but everyone can benefit from trigger point therapy, no matter how severe their symptoms are. Therapists in many cases use the process of elimination to determine what is going to work for each client.

Trigger Point Therapy

Trigger point therapy involves deep pressure and rubbing muscles along the direction of the muscle fibers. This is why seeing a professional with hands-on experience with trigger points is important. The anatomy of the muscles surrounding the trigger points is very complex, and the therapy requires the professional to find the particular muscles in order to relieve them. Although it is considered to be a trial-and-error therapy, a trained therapist can quickly find the right area to focus on.

Good therapy can be hard to find. Plenty of therapists consider themselves to be trigger point specialists. I encourage you to do your research. Thankfully, there are many people who have learned to treat their trigger points on their own. It can be difficult to learn how, but speak with your therapists about techniques you can do at home.

Painkillers are often prescribed, rather than taking an effort to combat the problem at the source with massage therapy.

A light massage can ease tension on or around the trigger points, though it cannot resolve them. People resort to various forms of alternative medicine, such as aromatherapy and chiropractic services.[18] Travell and Simons have written two volumes on trigger points. I have used these books for decades in treatment. What I like most about these books is that they have excellent diagrams, they teach how to eliminate the trigger points, and they review how to prevent pain by using specific exercises and habitual ADLs. Trigger point therapy is not considered to be a complete cure for pain associated with trigger points. It is simply a tool to incorporate to provide some relief and continue healing.

SELF-TREATMENTS

There are numerous treatments that someone can perform on themselves. Many of them can be free or have minimal costs involved, and the benefits can be worth the effort.

Tennis Ball on Butt

The tennis ball works surprisingly well as a tool to help relieve pain. Many physical therapists keep them around the clinic for this reason. I recommend keeping a tennis ball in a long tube sock, because if it should drop, it is much easier to pick up.

By placing a tennis ball under your butt to apply some pressure, blood is encouraged to resupply the muscles and fascia on the back of your hips. An easier way to do this is to roll your butt against a tennis ball next to the wall. Your backside comprises a very large set of muscles called the gluteals. The gluteal muscles are responsible for stabilizing the leg and hip socket, enabling you to stand upright. Massaging this area keeps muscle tissue supplied with fresh, oxygenated blood, which will contribute greatly to reducing lower back and sciatic pain.

Kinesiology Tape

Kinesiology tape is a new method of rehabilitation that is able to facilitate your body's natural healing process, with the added benefit of providing stability and support to joints and muscles.[19]

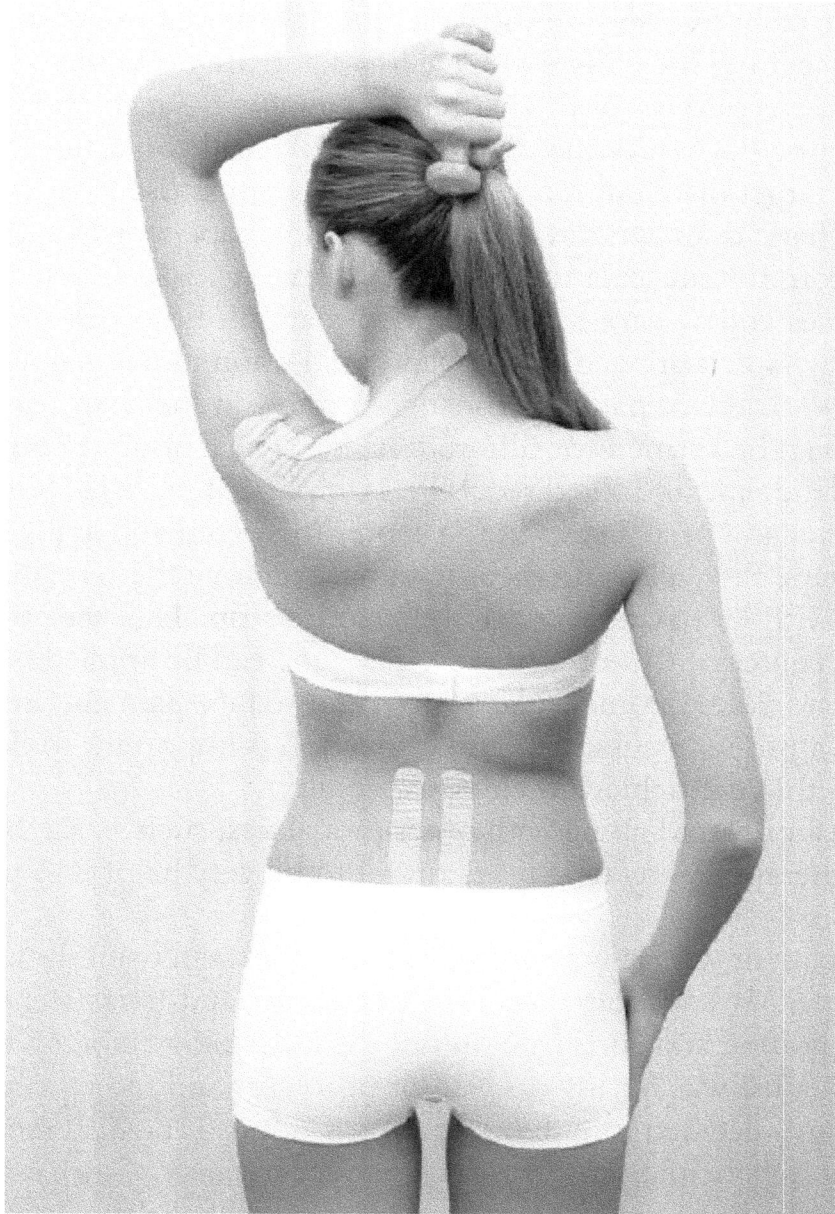

Benefits of Using Kinesiology Tape

Kinesiology tape is able to do all of this without restricting the body's range of motion in the way that many splints can. The tape is able to provide soft-tissue mobilization to prolong benefits after manual therapy. If I ever have an acute flare-up of back pain, I get a lot of relief from simply applying two strips of tape on my back (pictured above). My husband constantly asks for "the tape" on his back, knees, and shoulders!

You may have seen this tape before; it has become popular in recent years. Many people recognize this colorful tape worn by Olympians on television.

Many tapes are latex-free and can be worn for days at a time. As the tape begins to peel, simply cut off the ends that have lifted and are no longer sticky. Kinesiology tape is safe for both children and adults. It successfully treats a variety of orthopedic, neuromuscular, and neurological conditions. Kinesiology tape is able to target different receptors inside the somatosensory system to promote lymphatic drainage and alleviate pain. The tape works by lifting the skin slightly from the musculature below, allowing increased circulation of the interstitial spaces and a decrease in the inflammation of the affected areas.

Kinesiology tape is applied to the skin based upon individual needs. Strips are applied in a variety of patterns, most commonly in the shape of I, X, and Y. Other shapes can be formed for different needs. The amount of stretch during application of the tape and the direction it is applied are crucial. Some users find it preferable to tear a precut strip in the center to stretch and apply the exposed center of the tape first, allowing them to simply remove the remaining tag ends to tape down without having to stretch the entire strip. This way, there is only tension in the center of the strip of tape. The tape can be applied in countless way to reeducate the neuromuscular system and reduce pain and inflammation.

Receiving a proper assessment and evaluation is important to determine the style of taping that will achieve the desired results.

The tape can be used along with other modalities, such as ice, heat, or ML830 laser therapy. Many tape users find it to be very helpful to prevent injury as well.

Jessica, a patient who is very active, told me, "I wasn't sure how I felt about kinesiology tape. My back flared up four weeks ago, and I was feeling strong enough to go golfing and surfing. You put the kinesiology tape on my back the day before I went. I was having no pain or problems and the tape stayed on for two days before I decided to pull the rest off. I noticed the difference right away! The tape was helping my muscles contract because of its elasticity, making it easier to paddle. But I could only stand to golf another thirty minutes without the tape before I called it a day. I am back for more tape!"

Tape application can be tricky. The tape is applied over the affected area with the muscles extended, or stretched. The middle of the tape is also stretched before application, and the ends are left as is. This way, when the tape is applied, the mid-section of the tape has some tension to lift the skin from the muscle to increase circulation.

There are different colors available from a variety of brands. Most times, the color makes no difference, besides personal preference. However, many patients would seriously tell me, "Dr. Walker Gray, the pink works better than the black tape," or "The turquoise tape works best!" I would simply respond by saying, "I have heard that before!"

Here are some other suggestions for having success with kinesiology tape:

- Use an alcoholic wipe to remove any oil, sweat, or lotion that might be on the skin.

- After applying the tape, rub it on the outside to generate heat. The glue will become more adhesive.

- If you plan on getting the tape wet, be sure you have worn it for longer than one hour.

- Avoid stretching so far with the tape that it becomes detached or irritates the skin.

- Skin irritation is rare, but it should be monitored. If skin becomes irritated, remove tape immediately and rinse with cold water and soap. For sensitive skin, try applying milk of magnesia directly to the skin with a cotton ball. I like to apply the milk of magnesia and then use a hair dryer to dry it before reapplying the tape.

---

[16] Lynn A. Caruso, D. E. Chan, "Evaluation and management of the patient with acute back pain," *The American Journal of Occupational Therapy*, May 1986, doi.org/10.5014/ajot.40.5.347.

[17] Bente K. Pedersen, "Muscle as a secretory organ," *Comprehensive Physiology*, July 2013, vol. 3, no. 3, doi.org/10.1002/cphy.c120033.

[18] Janet G. Travell, D. G. Simons, *Myofascial Pain and Dysfunction: The Trigger Point Manual*, vols. 1 and 2, Philadelphia: Lippincott Williams and Wilkins, 1999.

[19] Lee Kwansub, "The effects of kinesiology taping therapy on degenerative knee arthritis patients' pain, function, and joint range of motion," *Journal of Physical Therapy Science*, January 2016.

Chapter 8

Solution Five:
Dietary Solutions versus Medications

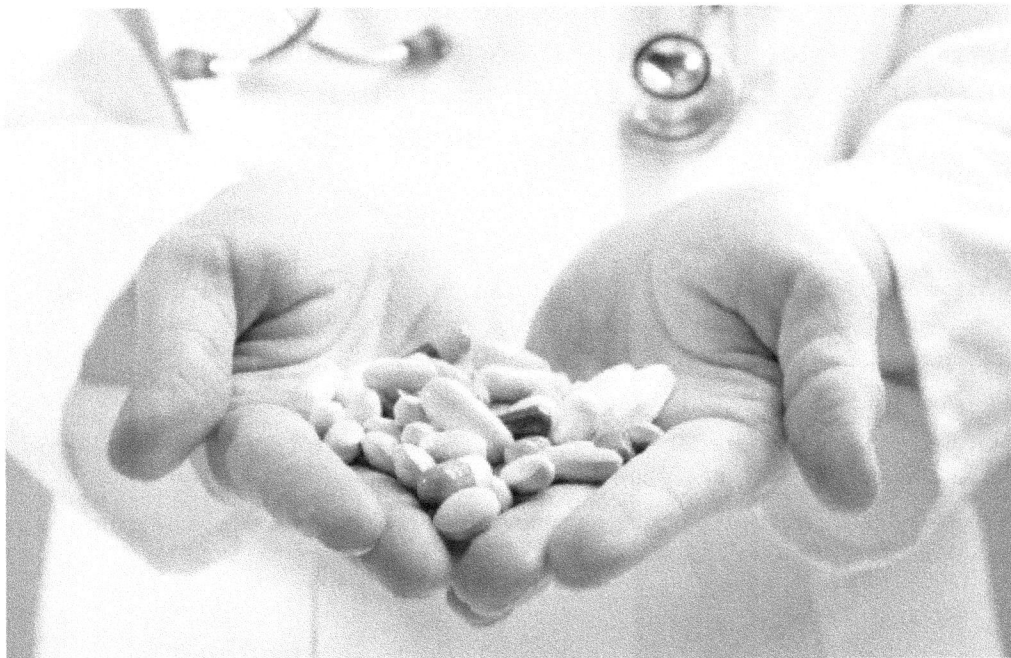

Depending on the level of pain that comes with low back pain and sciatica, some people need some type of pain relief. Many people take the easy route and take the pain relievers prescribed by their doctor. It is important to remember that some of these prescription pain relievers can be addicting and can also take a toll on your liver and kidneys. Furthermore, prescription and over-the-counter pain relievers are only good for masking problems. Sometimes pain relievers can be so effective, you might actually be causing more damage because you are unable to feel pain.

Prescription Painkillers

Today, typical medical treatment of low back pain and sciatica usually involves taking prescription painkillers with high risks of abuse and addiction. In 2016, the Centers for Disease Control and Prevention issued a revised recommendation for prescription guidelines to reduce the length of time someone takes painkiller prescriptions. Prescription painkillers are ineffective at treating the root cause of low back and sciatic pain.

In 2016, the *Journal of the American Medical Association*, a peer-reviewed medical journal, released a meta-analysis of twenty research studies concerning the use of opioids to treat chronic low back pain.[20] They found that opioids were only effective at treating modest short-term pain. None of the studies found significant pain relief following the use of prescription opioids.

The meta-study highlighted an interesting point concerning opioid studies: all the studies of opioid usage are short-term. There are very few high-quality studies that discuss the long-term effects of patients' using opioids for chronic low back pain. In a recent study patients with low back pain who took ibuprofen for a twelve-month period had the same amount of pain relief as those who took opioid medications, without the dangers of taking prescription opioid medications.[21]

In addition to offering minimal help to patients, opioid drugs can actually make chronic pain even worse. Some patients who use opioids can develop hyperalgesia, a paradoxical response whereby patients who consume these drugs become even more sensitive to painful stimuli.

Over-the-Counter Medications

Pain relievers generally fall into two categories: some treat inflammation, while others reduce pain. Non-steroidal anti-inflammatory drugs (NSAIDs) work to reduce inflammation. Inflammation is a problem for many people with low back pain and sciatica. Many people experience symptoms due to the inflamed tissue pushing on nerves and muscles from within. NSAIDs are not considered to be addictive and do not have psychoactive qualities. They are generally safe to use for short-term treatments. Long-term use of NSAIDs can cause damage to the liver and kidneys.

Pain relievers that are used to block pain signals in the brain are very addictive because of their psychoactive qualities. These medications are the opiates and opioids. They can be dangerous because they block important pain signals. For instance, if you choose to lie down in bed after taking a pain reliever, you might fall asleep in a position that is damaging and can cause pain and inflammation once you get up.

INJECTIONS

Epidurals

Epidurals are injections for back pain. They are injected directly into the area causing pain. The injections contain powerful anti-inflammatory steroids. The goal of the epidural is to reduce inflammation around the area that is causing pain.

Selective Nerve Root Block

Different from an epidural, a selective nerve root block (SNRB) is an injection of a cortisone steroid directly to the area causing pain. However, SNRBs do not target the inflammation surrounding a nerve, they target the nerve itself. The goal of an SNRB is to literally "numb" the nerve so it no longer sends painful messages to the brain.

Facet Injections

A facet-joint block is a minimally invasive procedure that involves a physician delivering a small amount of local anesthetic directly into the facet joint between vertebrae. Fluoroscopy (a real-time X-ray) is used to help guide the physician directly to the affected area. The purpose of the local anesthetic is to numb the pain in the area between the joints. Facet-joint blocks can be useful for reducing inflammation and providing long-term pain relief.

Discogram

A discogram is a test used to evaluate the structure of the vertebral column and help find the cause of back pain. During a discogram, dye is injected into the soft center of one or more vertebrae. The purpose of the dye is to identify any abnormal structures, such as cracks in a disc's exterior. The dye may show areas of wear and tear. Discograms are not normally performed until your doctor determines your pain to be chronic.

BETTER SOLUTIONS

The research is very clear: prescription opioids are not the primary solution for low back and sciatic pain; they are harmful and could make the pain worse. Holistic treatments—such as physical and occupational therapy, chiropractic treatment, exercise, diet, supplements, herbs, laser, CBD oil, meditation, and aromatherapy—are far more preferable and safe.

I was fortunate to study at the Natural Healing Institute in Encinitas, California. There, I became a certified clinical nutritionist (CCN) in 2011 and a certified clinical master of herbology in 2012 as part of my holistic-healthcare-practitioner certificate, obtained in 2013. This provided me with more holistic methods to help myself, my family, and my patients.

No one ever has pleasant thoughts about pain. However, it is important to know that your body produces pain signals for a reason. That is your body telling you to stop what you are doing!

Kathy R., a former patient and retired schoolteacher, said, "I used to have to take over-the-counter (OTC) anti-inflammatory medications every day after I exercised. After years of doing this, my doctor warned me that my liver might have complications from taking OTC medications for so long. I became worried and did my research. It took a few weeks to finalize a natural supplement plan, but I am happy to say I found a combination of herbs and supplements that provide greater relief than OTC medications ever could!"

DIET

Sound judgment will tell you that a healthy individual will recover more quickly from injury than someone whose diet consists of energy drinks and candy. A balanced consumption of vitamins and minerals will allow your body to perform at its peak. The basic plan of action to achieve health should be to focus on freshness and variety.

Prioritizing healthy eating habits will improve your body's ability to cope with the normal difficulties of everyday life. Eating healthily will raise your physical tolerance to stress and anxiety. Often a result of reduced stress is less sciatica and low back pain.

By choosing to eat healthily, you are also doing a service to your cardiovascular system. Blood pressure is undoubtedly affected by health and diet. Your circulatory system is essential for removing toxins and inflammation throughout the body. The benefits of eating more healthily not only reduce sciatica and low back pain but can also add years to your life!

What Excessive Weight Does to You

Excessive weight and surplus body fat have the benefit of keeping you warm during the cold season—and that's about where the benefits end. Surplus body fat is destructive to your spine. The lower vertebrae are more affected by body weight than the upper vertebrae are. This is why more overweight people than underweight people are affected by back pain. Even a few extra pounds hanging over the lower vertebrae force the body to work much harder than it would if the extra weight were not present.

Increased body weight can be particularly troublesome if you gain it in a short period of time. This is, of course, why many pregnant women develop low back pain due to the increase in forward weight and associated changes in center of gravity. The body has a very limited time during pregnancy to react to the increased weight gains. In cases of high weight gain in a small period of time, the effects of each extra pound are exponentially more strenuous on the low back, especially for an individual who is already lightweight.

Your Diet Can Help Diminish the Effects of Sciatica and Low Back Pain

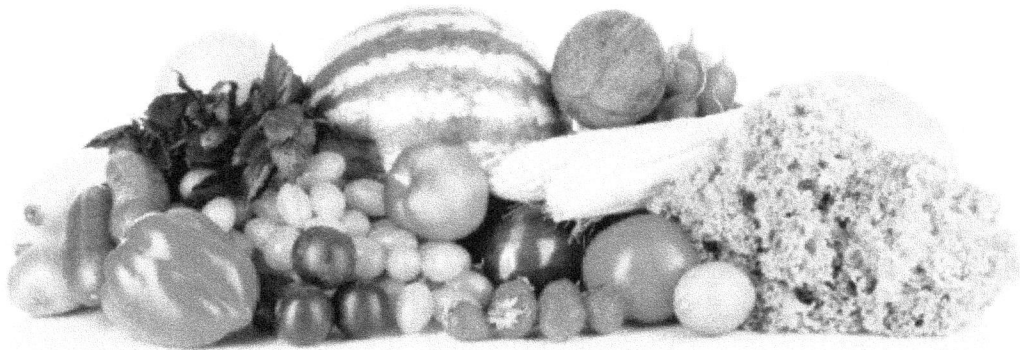

Most people are now well aware of the pain that sciatica and low back pain can cause. Many people are stunned the first time their doctor makes the link between physical pain and current health and diet status. It is a sobering moment!

Strong bones are important to avoid complications that can cause even more pain, such as arthritis and osteoporosis. If you suffer from osteoporosis, for example, an increase in calcium would benefit you. Be cautious of your alcohol intake, as it can reduce the amount of calcium your body is able to absorb. Knowledge is half the battle! It is important to know your body and work with professionals to find out what you are lacking. Taking on a healthy diet will allow you to live a more enjoyable, pain-free life.

Whether you are in the middle of combating sciatica or low back pain at this very moment or you just want to prevent these painful conditions, here are some ways experts have suggested to improve your diet. First and foremost, calcium is key to having strong bones. Although, recently, Japanese researchers have discovered something different that can help—making sure you have sufficient vitamin K.

It is assumed that vitamin K—found in broccoli, spinach, and other dark, leafy green vegetables—facilitates calcium retention inside the bones, helping to build strength and prevent injury. Strong bones are the foundation of strong bodies. Strong bodies are less likely to be affected by low back pain and sciatica. Strong bodies make faster recoveries, too.

My husband and I like to follow the anti-inflammatory diet, which is also known as the Mediterranean diet. We include natural fats in our meals and snacks (almond butter, avocados, and nuts), as well as whole-grain sprouted bread, steel-cut oatmeal, and organic fruits and vegetables.

I am not trying to bore you with the new healthy diet discoveries of last year. My aim is to educate you about some important dietary recommendations that have worked for me and my clients. I strongly recommend eating this nutrient-dense diet four times a day:

- 40 percent of calories from carbs with a low glycemic index,
- 30 percent of calories from protein, and
- 20 to 30 percent of calories from healthy fats.

A Practical Nutrient-Dense Diet

Patti Weller, CCN, author of *The Power of Nutrient Dense Food,* recommends a practical nutrient-dense diet of 1,800 calories, which should consist of these alternatives[22]:

- Dairy: 1 cup (c.) plain, nonfat yogurt; 1 c. 2% milk
- Fruits: 1 c. fresh blackberries; 1 c. orange slices; 1 c. cantaloupe
- Grains: 1 slice whole wheat bread (about 1.5 oz.)
- Legumes: ½ c. green peas; ½ c. mung beans (measured after cooking)
- Starchy vegetables: 1 small potato in its skin (1.5 oz., measured after cooking)
- Protein foods: 3 oz. top sirloin beef; 2 eggs; 3 oz. pink salmon (measured after cooking)
- Nuts, seeds, and oils: ½ oz. almonds; 1 tbsp. sunflower seeds; 1 tsp. flaxseed oil, ½ tbsp. butter
- Vegetables: 1 c. carrots; 1 c. red peppers; 1 c. spinach; ½ c. kale; 1 c. broccoli; 1 c. bok choy; ½ oz. dried shiitake mushrooms (measured after cooking)

Follow these general recommendations:

- Avoid all processed foods.
- Eat fresh, organic fruits and vegetables as much as possible. You may have to eat fruit as a snack in between meals if you find you cannot digest it well with other foods.
- Limit seafood to three times per week. Check for mercury content at GotMercury.org, "Calculator for Mercury in Fish."
- Limit animal protein to one portion of meat, seafood, or poultry per day. Eat other protein sources, like beans.
- Avoid all trans fats (fried foods) … except on rare occasions!
- Limit saturated fats to no more than once a week.
- Avoid most canned foods due to their high sodium content (exceptions are some canned seafoods; read the label).
- Eat only those frozen vegetables that are low in sugar and salt, with no added sauces.
- Limit frozen entrees to 400 mg of sodium, 7 g of sugar and 10 g of fat once a day.
- Avoid all foods with high-fructose corn syrup as an ingredient, as it may interfere with the body's ability to absorb and use copper.
- Sprinkle sea veggies on soups and salads.
- Introduce fermented veggies into your diet.
- Try to limit alcohol to an occasional glass of red wine.
- Drink between six and eight glasses of water per day.
- Avoid coffee. If you are a coffee drinker, it may take several weeks to quit. I would recommend that coffee drinkers cut their consumption in half the first week, half again the second week, and half again the third week. For the fourth week, switch to green or white tea.

Foods

Vegetables contain varying amounts of fiber and water, and some good fats. Their nutrients and phytonutrients will enrich your diet and assist with pain relief.[23] It is important to eat a variety of vegetables because each vegetable exhibits different nutrients.

- Artichokes (cooked) contain choline, folate, magnesium, vitamins B3 and K, copper, manganese, potassium
- Bok choy contains vitamin A, calcium, potassium

- Brussels sprouts contain vitamins C and K, choline, folate, potassium
- Butternut squash contains vitamins A, C, and E, magnesium, potassium, manganese
- Cabbage contains vitamins K, B6, and C, folate, chromium, manganese, calcium
- Carrots contain vitamins A, B1, B3, B5, B6, E, and K, biotin, boron, chromium, potassium
- Celery contains vitamin K, folate, calcium, potassium
- Garlic contains vitamin B6, copper, manganese, calcium
- Green beans contain folate, vitamin K, manganese
- Green peas contain vitamin B1, biotin, chromium, gamma tocopherol
- Green soybeans contain folate, vitamin K, manganese
- Kale contains vitamins A, B6, C, E, and K, copper, manganese, calcium
- Spinach contains vitamins A, B1, B2, B6, and E, chromium, copper, folate, magnesium, manganese, potassium, fiber, phosphorus, protein, zinc, choline
- Swiss chard contains vitamins A, E, and K, biotin, choline, copper, magnesium, potassium, sodium
- Turnip greens contain vitamins A, B6, C, E, and K, calcium, copper, manganese, folate
- Wheat germ contains vitamins B1, B2, B3, B5, B6, and E, magnesium, manganese, phosphorus, selenium, zinc, folate, iron, protein

A variety of fruits are rich in vitamins C and E, fiber, lycopene, copper, potassium, and manganese. Fruits are cleansing to the body, and this in turn decreases chronic pain. Fruits are a great supplement at each meal, in your cereal, or as a salad.

Eat fresh, organic fruits at the start of a meal or in between meals to allow the body to more easily digest and absorb the nutrients. Remember that fruits have sugars that, although natural, can affect sugar levels in diabetics. Just like with vegetables, it is important to eat a variety of fruits, because each fruit contains certain vitamins and minerals. If you are diabetic, take this list to your doctor or dietician to assess before adding them to your diet.

Below is a list of recommended fruits, showing the nutrients and micronutrients:

- Almonds contain vitamins E and B2, mono and polyunsaturated fats, copper, magnesium, fiber

- Apples contain boron, chromium, fiber
- Avocados contain vitamins B5, B6, and E, copper, fiber, biotin, boron, monounsaturated fats
- Bananas contain vitamin B6, biotin, copper, fiber, manganese, potassium
- Blackberries contain vitamins B5, C, E, and K, copper, gamma tocopherol, manganese, folate, magnesium, zinc, calcium, potassium
- Blueberries contain fiber, vitamin K, manganese
- Grapefruit, pink and red, contains vitamins A, B5, and C, fiber, potassium
- Medjool dates contain boron, copper
- Pomegranates contain fiber, copper, folate, potassium, vitamins C and K
- Valencia oranges contain vitamins B1, B5, and C, fiber, boron, chromium, folate, calcium, potassium

Additional supplements to aid in pain relief include the following:

- Vitamin B3: The niacinamide form should be taken with protein (no bread or crackers); however, B3 can also be taken in a complex (see below).
- Vitamin C: Start with 200 mg four times per day, and this can be increased to 600 mg. The powdered vitamin C is recommended and can either be sprinkled on food or mixed with water.
- Vitamin E: Recommended with meals or a glass of water.
- Boron
- Omega 3 fatty acids: Take with meals.
- Consider supplementing with ArthroSoothe, made by Designs for Health. This formula combines many of the vitamins and herbs mentioned above, and includes vitamin B3, zinc, selenium, copper, manganese, glucosamine sulfate, methylsulfonylmethane (MSM), N-Acetyl L-Cysteine (NAC), Boswellia resin (from *Boswellia serrata*), turmeric (*Curcuma longa*), cetyl myristoleate, hyaluronic acid, *Polygonum cuspidatum* (root), type II collagen, and microcrystalline cellulose, plus vegetable stearate, rice flour, and silicon dioxide. ArthroSoothe capsules be purchased from Amazon. I was introduced to this dietary supplement by an orthopedic surgeon who told me this was the best one he could find for his arthritic pains. ArthroSoothe recently added a pain-relieving cream to their product list. It contains glucosamine, sulfur (MSM), hyaluronic acid, arnica, chamomile, aloe vera, emu oil, and caprylic capric triglycerides from coconut.
- For arthritic pain relief, I was recently introduced to Vibrant Health's Joint

Vibrance powder by Gregory Smith, MD, who told me that he has effectively used this supplement, along with CBD oil, with his arthritic patients over the past ten years. Joint Vibrance contains everything good, including vitamin C, calcium, iron, magnesium, zinc, potassium, types I and II collagen, glucosamine, chondroitin, MSM (methylsulfonylmethane), Boswellia resin, bromelain, turmeric, hyaluronic acid, and silica from horsetail stem. It can be purchased at Amazon. Dr. Smith recommends getting the Joint Vibrance powder rather than the tablets, for enhanced absorbency, and to take two scoops a day with juice or water for one month to saturate your system, and then go to one scoop per day.

HERBS

Depending on the severity of your pain, you might need some type of external pain relief. Severe pain can get in the way of daily activities. It is important to find some relief, if necessary, to continue living an independent lifestyle.

Before taking herbs, always check with your medical doctor, as it is important to check your current medications to ensure there will be no adverse reactions. There are many excellent alternatives to "big pharma" medications. Most herbs do not have severe side effects like prescribed or over-the-counter medications. The use of the natural alternatives discussed here should always be presented to and monitored by your physician. Even natural herbs can have negative interactions with medications you must take.

Willow Bark

You might be surprised to learn that the main ingredient in aspirin, acetylsalicylic acid, is derived from the salicylic acid found in willow bark. The absorption rate is slower from willow bark, but there is evidence that maintaining a consistent dose for a week can bring pain relief. People who are affected by osteoporosis have also found pain relief from willow bark, without any side effects. If you are sensitive to aspirin, you will want to avoid willow bark.

Boswellia Trees

The resin from Boswellia trees has proven to be an excellent anti-inflammatory. A study conducted in 2011 by Ms. Raychaudhuri in India shows that the extract of the plant *Boswellia serrata* can reduce pain and considerably improve joint functions, in some cases providing relief even within seven days. More research needs to be done on Boswellia tree resin to show its true potential, but so far research looks very promising. Personally, I am a big fan of this herb and I put some in my tea in the mornings. My hormone doctor is also a fan of this herb.

Sour Cherries

Sour cherries have yet to be studied in depth, but current research is very positive. Sour cherries can inhibit the production of inflammatory enzymes, much like ibuprofen. Sour cherries have antioxidant qualities and are believed to be effective in reducing the rate of cancer growth as well.

Ginger

Recent research shows that increasing the amount of ginger you consume, naturally or via supplement, can relieve stiffness from osteoarthritis. The pain-relieving qualities of ginger are still not well understood, although it has been used as a pain reliever for thousands of years in different cultures around the world.

Nettles

Freeze-dried nettles are available in capsule form at Amazon. When nettles are in season I like to do a quick sauté with oil and garlic, or include it with whole-grain pastas or brown rice pilafs. Nettles are believed to help with pain associated with arthritis.

Turmeric

Turmeric is part of the ginger family. Its main ingredient is curcumin. A study conducted by Ms. Chainani-Wu confirmed that curcumin has strong anti-inflammatory qualities. It has been effective for reducing pain from rheumatoid arthritis, ulcerative colitis, osteoporosis, and fibromyalgia. Curcumin is not recommended for those suffering from hyperacidity, stomach ulcers, or gallstones.

CARLY'S DIET

"I used to eat so badly," said Carly, a former client. "I started to have low back pain and I wasn't sure where to start. I began physical therapy and wanted to change everything about my life. I began a recommended diet and found that I felt healthier. After a few months of eating this way, I began to lose weight. I was stronger from exercise. My back pain completely went away! My body had come full circle and I've kept it that way."

You are probably aware of the basic rules for healthy eating. This content should give you some new and exciting ideas about the foods and supplements to add to your diet without breaking the bank. If you need extra attention in this area, consult a dietician or nutritionist about how to make some simple, healthy changes to your diet.

Just think of your diet as preventive medicine. An improved diet can be easy to incorporate into your lifestyle—easier to incorporate than a walker or a cane, in the long run!

---

[20] Christina Abdel Shaheed, C. G. Maher, K. A. Williams, et al, "Efficacy, tolerability, and dose-dependent effects of opioid analgesics for low back pain: A systematic review and meta-analysis," *The Journal of the American Medical Association*, July 2016, doi.org/10.1001/jamainternmed.2016.1251.

[21] E. E. Krebs, A. Gravely, S. Nugent, et al, "Effect of opioid vs nonopioid medications on pain-related function in patients with chronic back pain or hip or knee osteoarthritis pain. The SPACE randomized clinical trial," *The Journal of the American Medical Association*, March 2018, doi.org/10.1001/jama.2018.0899.

[22] Patti Weller, *The Power of Nutrient Dense Food*, San Diego: Deerpath, 2014.

[23] Ibid.

Chapter 9

Solution Six: Aromatherapy

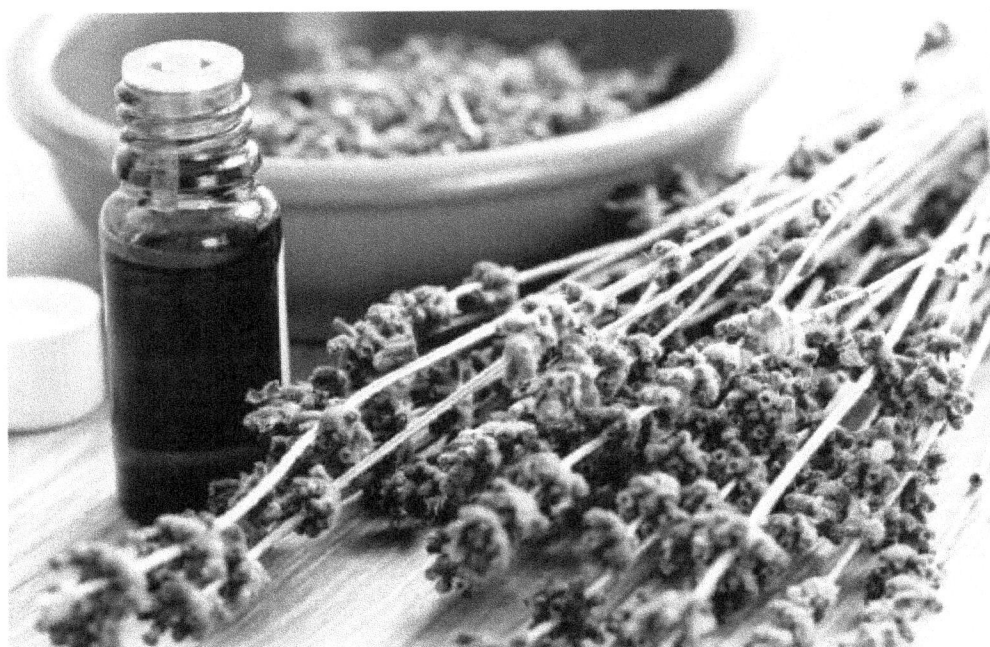

Back pain can ruin a perfect day, especially lower back pain. It can be difficult to lie down, stand up, and everything in between. Even driving the car can be aggravating.

Those of us who work behind a desk are more prone to low back pain and especially sciatica. Sitting for extended periods of time puts an incredible amount of stress on your back and hips. Every type of pain, from strains to arthritis, amounts to one thing: suffering.

Pain is miserable. Everyone agrees! Chronic pain that lasts more than six months, not only affects us physically, it also affects us mentally. Research shows that chronic pain leads to depression. When our mind and soul become affected by pain, it is time to think outside the box to find relief.

What Is Aromatherapy?

Aromatherapy, also referred to as *essential oil therapy*, is a type of holistic treatment that draws natural healing properties from certain plant extracts in order to heal both the body and mind. I feel fortunate that I became a certified aromatherapist from the Natural Healing Institute of Naturopathy in Encinitas, California, in 2013. Aromatherapy has existed for thousands of years, dating back to ancient cultures throughout Asia and Egypt. More recently, it has gained support from Western scientific and medical communities.

A former client, June M., said, "I was hesitant to try aromatherapy to help with pain. I just wasn't sure it was going to work for my low back pain. I tried a few recommendations with an open mind. I found that it not only helped calm me to reduce my pain but it also helped me reduce the severity and duration of my migraine headaches."

While aromatherapy might sound far-fetched as a healing agent, it has gained more acceptance as new research emerges. From a scientific standpoint, it is believed that certain aromas work to stimulate smell receptors in the nose. These receptors then send messages through the nervous system to the limbic system, which is responsible for controlling our emotions.[24] Our local communities all have their own wonderful aromas, but they are limited. Have you ever felt the rush of serotonin from taking a hike after the rain, or from coming off an airplane into a luscious tropical region? These are the feelings that aromatherapy can provide.

Lakham, Sheafer, and Tepper in 2016 did a thorough study entitled "The Effectiveness of Aromatherapy in Reducing Pain: A Systemic Review and Meta-Analysis." They found that aromatherapy can successfully treat pain when combined with conventional treatment.[25]

Many people do not want to take medications to ease their low back pain and prefer natural methods. Essential oils such as lavender, marjoram, frankincense, and sweet ginger not only ease the pain but also induce relaxation. In order to enjoy the benefits of the essential oils and plant extracts used over the course of an aromatherapy treatment, individuals can use a variety of methods, such as diffusers, facial steamers, hot and cold compresses, baths, and topical applications, to name only a few. Common benefits of aromatherapy treatments range from pain management to enhanced quality of sleep.

Of course, you always want to check with a certified herbalist, aromatherapist, or doctor before using essential oils. It is important to be sure you will have no allergic reactions upon consuming any new substance.

During the day, I like using citrus essential oil. I mix ten drops of essential oil to one ounce jojoba oil. I will apply it two to three times a day to my ears and nose. Oil can also be applied to a light bulb or a diffuser. I may use lemon, orange, or grapefruit. If you use citrus oils on your skin, be sure to stay out of the sun—citrus oils can contain photosensitizers, which can cause serious skin damage, such as redness, burns, or blisters, when exposed to the sun.

Pain Relief Without a Prescription

Lower back pain can be mild or severe. Everyone also perceives pain differently. Those affected by severe pain are often advised to take over-the-counter medications and painkillers. As you previously read, pain relief in the form of such medications often carries the consequences of adverse side effects such as liver or kidney damage. It's safe to say that there are many forms of safer pain relief, and aromatherapy is at the top of the list!

Added Benefits of Aromatherapy

There are many added benefits to using essential oils for pain. Some people who find themselves anxious or depressed because of their chronic pain find relief from using essential oils.

Sleep issues, whether or not they are caused by pain, may also be alleviated with the use of the correct oils. A study from the journal *Evidence-Based Complementary Alternative Medicine* concluded that aromatherapy was effective in reducing the anxiety levels and increasing the sleep quality of patients admitted to the intensive care unit of a hospital.

WHICH ESSENTIAL OILS WORK FOR LOW BACK AND SCIATIC PAIN?

Eucalyptus Oil

Eucalyptus essential oil is one of the most commonly used oils to treat aches and pains. Eucalyptus oil has strong anti-inflammatory properties that work best when diluted into a carrier oil and used in massage. It can also be inhaled from a nebulizing essential oil diffuser. A quick Amazon search can lead you to choosing the right nebulizer; there are always improved models being released.

If you prefer topical solutions, it is suggested to use eucalyptus oil as a lotion for massage over sore or painful areas. It can be used to help treat nerve pain, aches, and sprains.

Lavender Oil

Lavender essential oil is by far one of the most popular oils used in a variety of products. Lavender oil has many uses and can treat a range of ailments. Lavender is a well-known anti-inflammatory. It is not irritating to the skin in the way that over-the-counter anti-inflammatory creams might be. Its pleasant aroma is known to reduce stress and increase sleep.

At night, my husband and I like lavender essential oil for relaxing and getting a good night's sleep. We grow English lavender in our yard. I dry it and crush it and put it into a little pillow for our bed. Also, before sleep, we dab a little lavender essential oil on our earlobes and under our noses, and frequently rub a little on our feet.

Frankincense Oil

Frankincense oil originates from the sap of the cut bark of the Boswellia tree. It has been used in beauty products for the skin for as long as there have been skin care products. This oil has a very relaxing aroma and can help ease tension when used in a nebulizing diffuser.

Sweet Ginger Oil

Sweet ginger essential oil is well known for being a natural cure for nausea. Nausea or vertigo can often accompany chronic pain that stems from the lower back or sciatica. Sweet ginger essential oil works best to reduce muscle soreness when it is diluted with a carrier oil and used topically. It can also be inhaled through a nebulizing diffuser.

Marjoram Oil

Marjoram essential oil is well known for its antispasmodic properties to soothe low back and sciatic pain. It works by calming muscles that have been fatigued and may have become tight or achy. Marjoram oil has a pleasant aroma that many find to be calming.

Chamomile Oil

Chamomile is one of the oldest and most popular herbs to make tea and oil from. Chamomile is an herb in the daisy family. It can be consumed in tea, applied topically to the skin, or inhaled in a nebulizer. It is known for its calming effects. It is also said to relieve digestive issues, reduce inflammation, and increase heart health. Chamomile has also been known to reduce allergy symptoms.

HOW TO USE ESSENTIAL OILS

For Painful Back Joints and Muscles

For myself personally, I have found a combination of turmeric, sage, and wintergreen essential oils combined with jojoba oil to be particularly effective for my painful back joints and muscles. For a four-ounce bottle, use 48 drops of turmeric, 48 drops of wintergreen, and 24 drops of sage. Fill the rest of the bottle with jojoba oil. Apply a dab of this oil to painful areas two to four times every day.

Before You Start

The first time you use essential oils, be sure to use only a minimal amount. Although all of the mentioned essential oils are natural, some people are allergic to some specific oils. Make sure that you have no allergies to them. Don't hesitate to consult your medical doctor about any possible allergies you may have.

Using essential oils in carrier oils for topical application or with massage is one of the most popular ways to deliver aromatherapy. A few carrier oils that are popular are sweet almond oil, apricot kernel oil, coconut oil, and jojoba oil (my personal favorite). After you find which essential oils work for you, consider taking your mixture to your massage therapist or physical therapist to be used during massage treatments.

Only a few drops of your chosen aromas are necessary—a little bit goes a long way. If you feel you need to increase or decrease the potency of the oil, feel free to experiment. Just remember, most essential oils for purchase are concentrated and should last a long time. After opening a bottle of essential oil, it is best to keep it in the fridge.

Other Forms of Aromatherapy

Some other aromas that are worth a mention are laurel, pine, rosemary, and valerian. These all have anti-inflammatory properties and very calming scents. Many of these essential oils will work topically. They can also be used in a warm bath.

Although salt might not fall under the topic of aromatherapy, warm baths with sea salts or Epsom salts are effective in reducing inflammation. Salt baths are also thought to change the body's pH levels, to allow absorption and elimination of different chemicals within the body. The next time you decide to take a bath, consider adding one or two cups of sea salt or Epsom salts. You may be surprised by the result.

Be sure that you are well hydrated when trying new aromatherapies. It is not uncommon to feel increased pain or limited reactions to aromatherapy because you are simply dehydrated. Aromatherapy is known for its simplicity and minimal side effects. It can be fun to seek out different oils. The effects can be subtle at first, but once you spend time *with* your chosen aromas, you won't want to go *without* them!

---

[24] Kathi Keville, Mindy Green, *Aromatherapy: A Complete Guide to the Healing Art*, New York: Crossing Press, 2008.

[25] Shaheen Lakhan, H. Sheafer, D. Tepper, "The effectiveness of aromatherapy in reducing pain: A systematic review and meta-analysis," *Pain Research and Treatment*, November 2016, doi.org/10.1155/2016/8158693.

Chapter 10

Solution Seven: ML830 Low-Level Laser

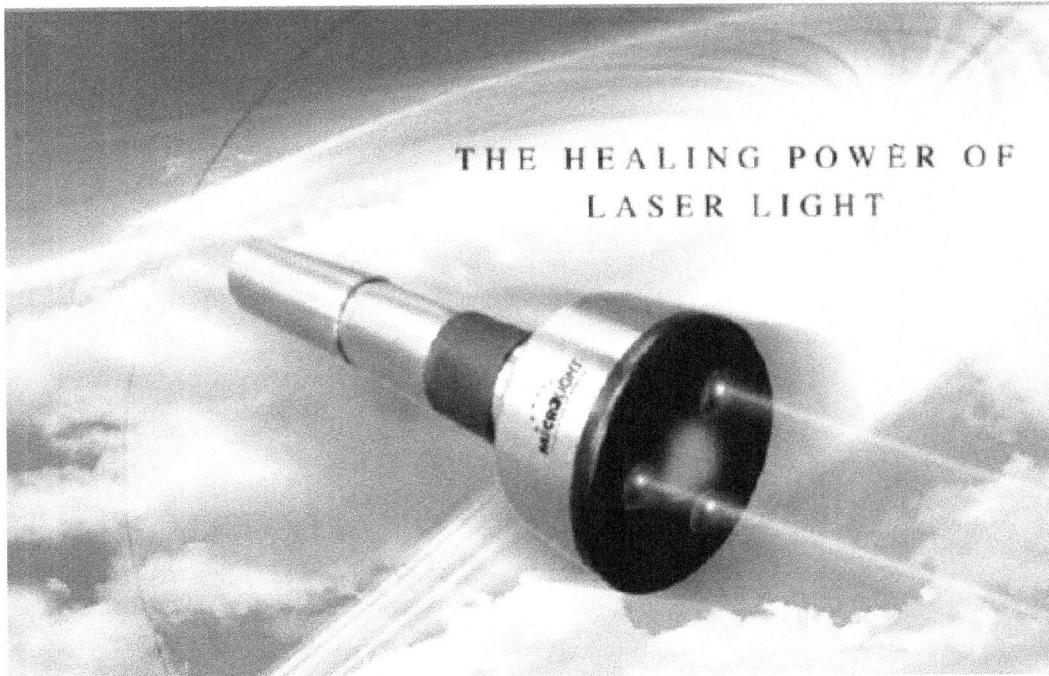

I want to share with you my cold-laser trip! In 2008, I attended a three-day seminar for physical and occupational therapists. We had the opportunity to learn about advanced practice techniques, services, and secrets to provide our clients with greater pain relief.

One secret I had learned about was the ML830 low-level laser. I was skeptical at first because we used a different laser in our clinic, which we found to be ineffective. My consultant said, "Grace, this laser is *different*, you *need* it!"

I contacted Michael Barbour, the owner and patent holder of the ML830 low-level laser. He offered to come to my practice within a week and teach my therapists how to operate the ML830 low-level laser. Michael is the founder of the Houston Laser Institute. He has proven to be exceptionally knowledgeable concerning cold laser treatment for pain and inflammation. His laser is FDA-approved since 2002 for the treatment of pain and inflammation.

The next Monday morning Michael was at my clinic. After signing consent forms, each of my toughest patients with low back and sciatic pain lined up to receive one complementary ten-minute sessions with the laser.

The results were astonishing! I made sure to have patients bend forward before and after their treatment with the laser to measure not only their pain levels but also how far they were able to bend forward. After the application of the laser I found that 80 percent to 85 percent of patients showed improvement in their ability to bend forward, and they reported less pain. Wow, was I impressed!

My husband was one of those who came in for a laser treatment session. He is in the legal profession, extremely analytical, judgmental, and basically a no-nonsense type of person. He is athletic and has experienced injuries from basketball and tennis. We applied the laser to his low back for a ten-minute treatment. Later at home, he said "It's unbelievable, Grace, the pain is gone!" He frequently asked me to bring the laser home on the weekends! I finally bought one for home use!

The ML830 low-level laser is a diode laser. Its continuous wavelength is of 830 nanometers (nm)—a billionth of one meter and has an output of 30 milliwatts (mW) at each of the three apertures, for a total of 90 mW. This laser belongs to the class III-B, which means that the direct beam is dangerous for direct eye contact. As a protective measure, patients are asked to wear appropriate goggles that protect their eyes against 800 to 850 wavelength spectrums.

SO, WHAT GETS BETTER FASTER WITH THE LASER?

What gets better faster with the laser? Every pain issue in muscles, ligaments, tendons, and joints through dysfunction. The laser also relieves inflammation, as well as aids in tissue regeneration. It is extremely effective with sciatica, slipped discs, and backache. Many times, in my practice, giving the laser prior to physical therapy treatment allowed tissue to respond better to stretching, trigger point releasing, and physical exercises. The laser is also extremely effective with scars and incisions after surgery.

My clinic's top joint-pain programs focused on the shoulders, neck, back, and knees. However, we also treated the jaw, elbows, wrists, hands, carpal tunnel disorders, hips, ankles and foot pain problems. We provided physical therapy programs for arthritis, fibromyalgia, temporomandibular joint (TMJ), neck pain, shoulder pain, knee pain, and back pain. We effectively added laser treatment sessions with our patients. In many cases, giving the laser prior to treatment resulted in tissue that was easier to mobilize and stretch and that responded to trigger point releases more easily.

I still remember Mary Anne, an eighty-five-year-old patient with a wonderful Texan drawl. "Dr. Walker Gray, I just loovve that laser! It's just like a magic wand!"

Another patient, Roberta, decided that she did not want to have the laser as part of her treatments. After several therapy sessions, I noticed she was not getting better. Before coming to physical therapy, she experienced lumbar spine facet complication, which is a painful condition affecting how the joints of each vertebrae move against one another. I said, "Roberta, today I want to give you a laser session before I treat you." I put the cone on the end of the laser to concentrate the waves' focal point, in this case, at the left side of one particular lumber facet.

Roberta was amazed by her reduced pain! The next time she came in and told me, "Dr. Walker Gray, do you really think it was the laser that made a difference?"

I said, "Yes, I do!"

Another patient, Shirley, came to my practice with a stiff, painful back. She decided to purchase nine laser treatment sessions to complement her physical therapy program. She was an enthusiast about her treatment, including the ancillary laser sessions. After her sixth session, she wrote a thank you card to her referring doctor: "Thank you for referring me to Walker Physical Therapy and Pain Center. The therapy and the laser are both wonderful!"

THE HEALING MECHANISM

The mechanism by which the laser affects cells is not well understood, but it seems to be based on biostimulation: the low-level radiation is absorbed by intracellular photoreceptors in the membrane of the mitochondria. The effects include a reduction in pain due to increased endorphins, a reduction in inflammation by way of reducing interleukin and C-reactive protein, and a tissue healing effect as a result of increased neovascularization and beneficial macrophage activity.

The ML830 low-level laser has been included in numerous research articles and journals proving its effectiveness. A study was done by Bruce Gundersen, DC. Dr. Gundersen found that, under a controlled protocol for specific pain, relative to a variety of conditions, the ML830 low-level laser can produce a consistent remission of pain perception in both acute and chronic situations.[26]

Another clinical trial conducted by Trevor Berry, DC, and Mark Burdorf, DC, found that the low-level laser "has the potential benefit for providing an effective means of reducing low back pain that is simple, quick, noninvasive, and side-effect free."[27]

Another study in Australia conducted by G. E. Djavid, MD, PhD, showed that in chronic low back pain, low-level laser therapy combined with exercise is more beneficial than exercise alone in the long run. This was a randomized trial.[28]

Bernard Filner, M.D, wrote a study entitled "Low-level Laser Therapy - a Clinician's View" that shows how effective the ML830 laser is for trigger points versus injecting them.[29] He contends that the laser inactivates trigger points. My experience is a patient definitely seem to prefer the laser over having an injection. This doctor has been instrumental in my education of using the ML830 low-level laser with my patients.

Michael Barbour holds the patent for all lasers in production between 800 and 900 nm. His patented ML830 low-level laser is used to treat pain, inflammation, and tissue healing. I have investigated other cold lasers on the market. The ML830 low-level laser is the least expensive on the market, with the best customer service. I once had an issue with my unit (which was being run daily for eight hours!). Before I could send it in for service, the manufacturer had already sent me a loaner to use so I wouldn't interrupt patient care. Good customer service is rare these days!

To find a practitioner close to you who uses the ML830 low-level laser go to https://microlightcorp.com/find-a-doctor/.

To purchase a laser, go to www.drgracewalkergray.com.

---

[26] Bruce Gundersen, "A clinical trial on low level laser therapy as a pain control modality," *The Academy of Chiropractor Orthopedists*, September 2005.

[27] Trevor Berry, Mark Burdorf, "Study of low level laser therapy to treat low back pain," *National Library of Medicine*, September 2014.

[28] G. E. Djavid, R. Mehrdad, M. Ghasemi, H. Hasan-Zadeh, A. Sotoodeh-Manesh, G. Pouryaghoub, "In chronic low back pain, low level laser therapy combined with exercise is more beneficial than exercise alone in the long term: A randomised trial," *Australian Journal of Physiotherapy*, 2007, doi.org/10.1016/S0004-9514(07)70022-3.

[29] Bernard Filner, "Low-level laser therapy-a clinician's view," *Practical Pain Management*, 2006, https://www.practicalpainmanagement.com/treatments/complementary/lasers/low-level-laser-therapy-clinician-view

Chapter 11

Solution Eight: Cannabidiol Oil

Cannabidiol oil (CBD oil) is destined to be a positive medical revelation! What's in cannabis that makes it a healing agent?

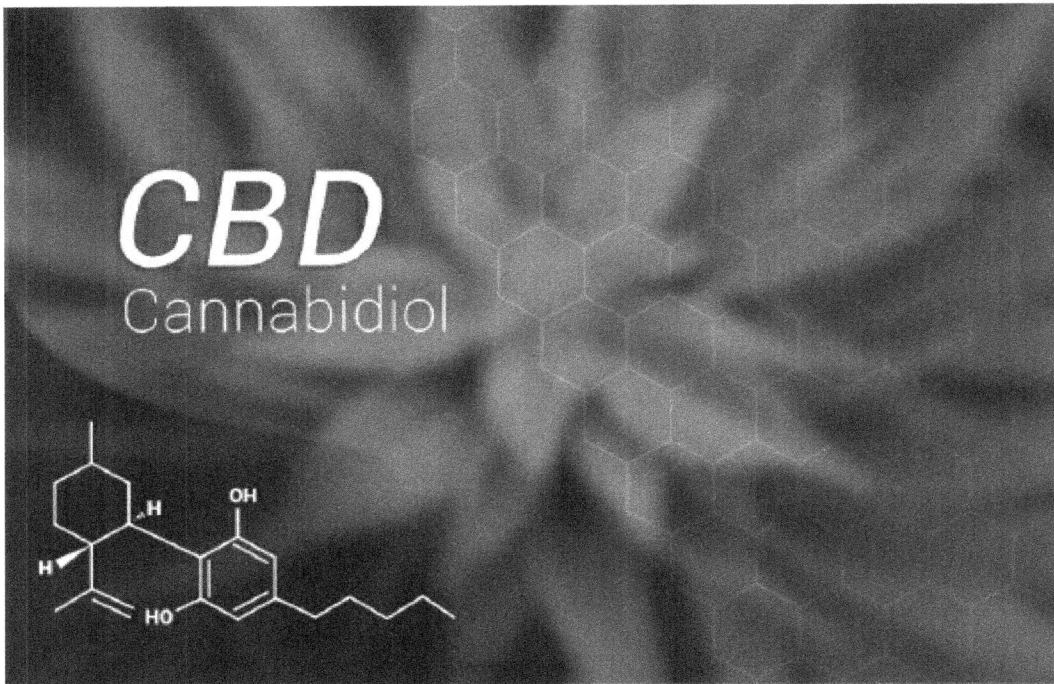

    Cannabis sativa, or cannabis, contains over 500 naturally occurring compounds. Many of these are called cannabinoids. Two of the natural compounds include cannabidiol (CBD) and tetrahydrocannabinol (THC). THC is the psychoactive component that makes one feel "high," whereas CBD has no psychoactive properties. CBD is typically derived from hemp, which has an extremely low content of THC.

    Although hemp and marijuana come from the same plant genus, they are actually different plants. Hemp is a different strain of the *Cannabis sativa* plant. For federal legality, CBD products must contain less than 0.3 percent THC. However, hemp naturally can have more than 3 percent. Hemp is used to make CBD products such as clothing, paper, building materials, foods, and even cosmetics. In 2018 the Farm Bill passed, allowing the cultivation of hemp at a federal level. The 2018 Farm Bill made it federally legal to grow hemp, even though some select states still do not allow CBD consumption. This bill allows the shipping of hemp and hemp-derived products (less than 0.3 percent THC) across state lines, and it also made it possible for farmers who grow hemp to get crop insurance, which had been a huge barrier to growing it prior to 2018.

As of July 2019, ten states have legalized cannabis to be grown and bought in small amounts, and there are three states (Nebraska, South Dakota, and Wyoming) with restrictions for *all* cannabis-derived products, including hemp and CBD. CBD's new status has not allowed enough time for researchers to understand the full benefits of CBD.[30] However, new research and studies are currently underway in the United States and abroad.

CBD's Interaction With the Body

The endocannabinoid system (ECS) in our body is a neuromodulator system. It consists of the cannabinoid receptors, CB1 and CB2, the endocannabinoids, and the enzymes that break down the cannabinoids. We humans have endocannabinoid receptors in our nervous system, brain, and nerve endings. CB1 receptors, located within the brain, interact with THC to make one feel high. We also have CB2 receptors throughout all our peripheral body systems.

Activation of the endocannabinoid system along with other supplements like ashanti pepper (different from black pepper) leads to homeostasis. A board-certified neurologist, Etan Russo, MD, coined the term *endocannabinoid deficiency syndrome.* When the body is deficient in receptors for cannabinoids, many health problems can arise, and symptoms can include chronic pain, arthritis, inflammation, depression, and autoimmune disorders. At this time, testing for the levels of endocannabinoids in our bodies is cost-prohibitive, so the clinical history and response to CBD is how we can gauge the efficacy of CBD or determine whether a different preparation is needed.

CBD is a natural anti-inflammatory. Using medical-grade CBD is much safer than using over-the-counter or prescription medications. Very few people experience side effects from CBD when compared to over-the-counter medications. CBD is safe to use. Recently, more and more respected medical professionals are starting to catch on as well.

Ever since CBD has been recognized for its therapeutic effects, there have been promising studies that show evidence that you may also find pain relief from CBD. Doctors at the University of Kentucky College of Medicine found that CBD gel applied directly to the joints of animals with arthritis for four days yielded greater range of motion.[31] Doctors in Germany found that CBD is helpful in subduing the fight-or-flight response that is activated with chronic inflammation. The nervous system terminals are controlled by CB1 receptors. Cannabinoids were found to modulate the receptor channels located on sensory nerve fibers, demonstrating how CB1 receptors affect arthritic pain.[32]

CBD oil can be ingested in a capsule. If you decide to take it orally, be sure you have food in your stomach. Many people with low back pain prefer the pain-relieving CBD lotion. CBD lotion can be applied directly over the area that is experiencing pain. It works by attaching to the body's pain receptors and works to dampen their signal. As CBD begins to build up in the system, the cycle of inflammation can be broken and reduce inflammation. Since CBD reduces the inflammatory response, swelling and stiffness of the joint are decreased.

My introduction to CBD came from a patient whose husband suffered from a degenerative neurological disorder. Her husband had been on opioid painkillers for nearly a decade before he tried CBD capsules. After taking CBD orally twice a day for only a week, he was able to reduce his painkiller consumption by 50 percent. Then, after doubling his CBD dosage, he was able to come off painkillers completely.

I was only exposed to CBD oil during my last year of owning my physical therapy clinic. I was amazed by CBD's ability to enhance treatment. Most clients preferred to use CBD topically as a lotion over affected areas. Using CBD as a topical lotion allows it to work quickly in relieving localized pain and inflammation directly over a joint or muscle.

I have not met anyone who has had negative interactions with CBD oil, whether or not they are taking prescription medications. Nevertheless, anyone who is considering taking CBD oil must notify their doctor first. Some doctors who choose to avoid research concerning CBD might not approve of it. It would be wise to consider a second opinion if your doctor is unwilling to review recent research.

People have used CBD oil for centuries to treat pain, but only lately has the medical community begun to truly study it. Many patients have found relief from their arthritis, sciatica, and low back pain using CBD. It also allows them to recover from their treatment programs with ease.

You want to be able to check the CBD you purchase. Is it a broad-spectrum product? In other words, does it include mainly CBD along with other cannabinoids, with no THC? Is it a full-spectrum product that contains terpenes, cannabinoids, flavonoids, and fatty acids found in hemp, all of which have their own therapeutic value? Has the product been third-party tested for purity and potency and can you review the lab sheets? Is the CBD free of solvents, pesticides, metals, and unnatural products? How do you feel when taking the products? If you ask these questions and do a little bit of research, you will probably dismiss many of the companies selling CBD oil online.

THE REAL PROBLEM WITH CBD TODAY

The current issue with CBD is that there is very little regulation of CBD products. Right now, there are many ineffective, impotent, junk CBD products on the market. Companies whose only goal is financial gain are producing low-quality CBD products. Some products that are being sold to treat medical illnesses were made in someone's garage or basement. Other CBD products are being mass-produced in China and shipped over to the US to be sold for profit. These products will not work! They are impure and lack quality control.

To make things worse, companies that sell CBD products are marketing them with misleading and inaccurate claims. Relying on false claims can be dangerous for people who need serious medical intervention. This type of marketing has given CBD a bad name in medical and political sectors. However, more research *is* developing. More testimonials are coming in demonstrating the benefits of CBD to help relieve pain for low back pain and sciatica.

THE BOTTOM LINE

The quality of CBD can vary widely. It is important you do your research to find the best quality products available to you. Many people respond well to CBD. It is very safe, even when taken in large doses.

Find a physician to monitor your use of CBD while you take prescription medications, especially if you have a serious illness. CBD is hemp-derived and does *not* require a prescription in most states. Hemp is not considered to be medical marijuana, since its THC (psychoactive component) content is less than 0.3 percent. CBD does not make people high, although some pain relief in itself can create quite a euphoric feeling! If you feel you have tried CBD and not had any relief, you may simply be taking too low a dose. A low dose could be totally ineffective, but a larger dose could yield great benefits. Be patient while you find the right dose.

Pregnant women and mothers who are breastfeeding should not take CBD.

A PERSONAL EXPERIENCE

Fortunately, a few years ago, I had the chance to meet Gregory A. Smith, MD, founder of Red Pill Medical, Inc. Dr. Smith came to my clinic and gave me and my therapists an informative session about CBD oil and products. I researched his products and found they met my criteria.

The products are broad-spectrum, and they have been third-party tested for purity and potency; I was personally able to review the lab sheets. I checked out Dr. Smith's CBD products and found they are free of solvents, pesticides, metals, and unnatural products. When I used the pain relief cream on my husband, patients, and myself, we all felt better! You can find many CBD products, including pain relief creams, capsules, essential oils, and supplements to achieve a certain effect, such as reduced pain and inflammation, sleep, and even weight control.

Ever since I was introduced to high-quality CBD products, I have had a bottle of pain relief cream on my bedside table for my husband and me to use. I practice what I preach, and take CBD capsules daily to activate my endocannabinoid system.

For more information on my recommended CBD products, go to my webpage, www.drgracewalkergray.com.

---

[30] Gregory Smith, *The Essentials of CBD*, self-pub., CreateSpace, 2017.

[31] D. C. Hammel, L. P. Zhang, F. Ma, S. M. Abshire, S. L. McIlwrath, A. L. Stinchcomb, K. N. Westlund, "Transdermal Cannabidiol reduces inflammation and pain-related behaviours in a rat model of arthritis," *The European Journal of Pain*, July 2016.

[32] T. Lowin, "Cannabinoid-based drugs targeting CB1 and TRPV1, the sympathetic nervous system and arthritis," *Arthritis Research & Therapy*, September 2015.

Chapter 12

Solution Nine:
Mindfulness

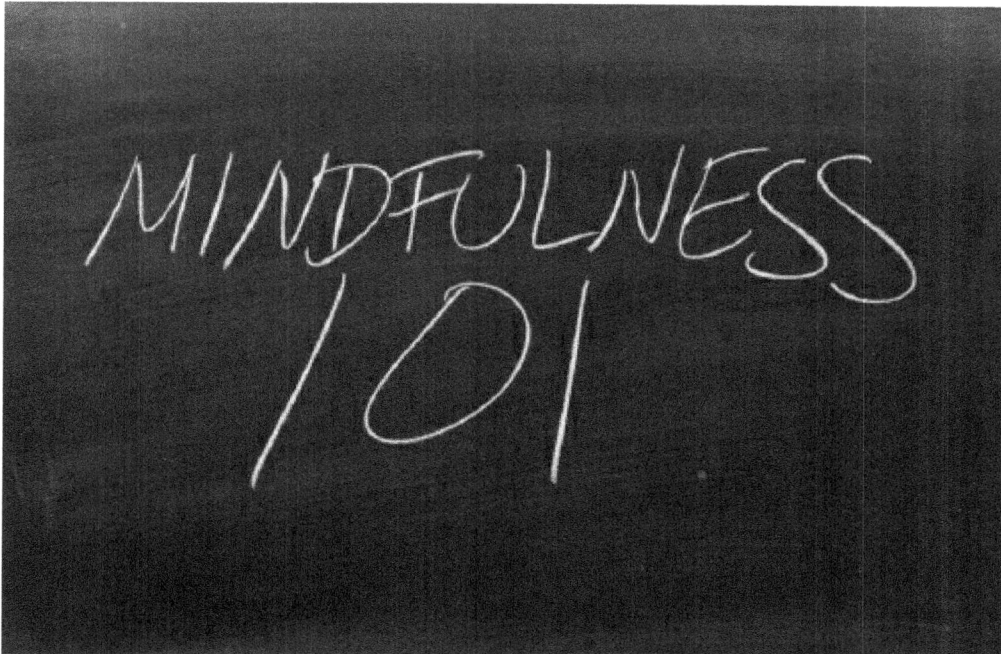

Jon Kabat-Zinn, PhD, began utilizing a 2,500-year-old Buddhist "insight" form of meditation to heal mental and physical illness. He began teaching these practices from a major New England teaching hospital over thirty years ago. Dr. Kabat-Zinn removed the religious and cultural aspects from the meditation and developed a method called *mindfulness-based stress reduction* (MBSR). MBSR is now taught all over the globe in a variety of settings, such as hospitals, medical schools, law schools, cancer centers, and major corporations.[33]

My studies as an occupational therapist taught me the importance of using this method to teach my clients and help them achieve more relief. MBSR is a type of meditation designed to help us acclimate to the present moment and be able to observe and accept our inner and outer experiences with greater compassion and patience. In the textbook *Pedretti's Occupational Therapy: Practice Skills for Everyday Functions* (eighth edition), chapter 7, there is a section written by occupational therapists (OTs) Pamela Richardson and Rochelle McLaughlin, which outlines the role of the OT using mindfulness in a treatment strategy for handling pain.[34]

Studies show that mindfulness meditation is a highly effective means of relieving chronic back pain.[35] One study in particular highlighted findings that mindfulness meditation was proven to increase activity in the areas of the brain that regulate emotion and decrease activity in the regions associated with pain.[36]

Although you can find yoga and meditation instructors who specialize in meditation, it is not too difficult to practice on your own. Continue reading to discover my top three fundamental mindfulness techniques that you can try on your own. They will not only alleviate low back and sciatic pain, they will increase your overall quality of life!

BODY SCAN MEDITATION

The point of this exercise is simply to notice your body. It is not only about relaxing your body; however, this may happen naturally. Typically, our response to pain is to either distract ourselves or focus on the area in pain. In this activity, you will notice and accept your pain with gentle curiosity.

Begin in a seated position or lying down. Ensure that you do not feel constricted, and loosen any tight clothing.

1. Begin with your feet, noticing the physical sensations in them: any discomfort, pain, warmth, cold, tension, tightness—anything. Don't interpret the sensations as good or bad. Don't try to change how they feel. Just be aware of them.

2. Slowly allow your awareness to rise from your feet up to your ankles and then your calves. How do your lower legs feel? Notice any pain or discomfort. Or perhaps there is no pain. Maybe your lower legs feel cool because it is breezy outside.

3. Slowly allow your awareness to drift up even further to your knees, and next to your thighs and hips, and so on. Identify how each part of your body is feeling at this moment. Continue on to your lower back, mid-back, stomach, chest, shoulders, upper arms, forearms, fingers, hands, neck, jaw, and head.

4. Let your consciousness drift gently and slowly back down your body, noticing other places where there is pain or discomfort. Simply notice how you are feeling in each part of your body, until your awareness settles back

down at your feet.

Practice doing this activity for five minutes. Don't worry about exactly how long this practice takes. Allow yourself to notice the different sensations in different parts of your body. If negative thoughts begin to intrude your practice, it's okay. Just notice your thoughts, and breathe. Let your abdomen rise and fall as you breathe in through your nose and out from your mouth. Gently guide your awareness throughout your body.[37]

MINDFUL BREATHING

Anxiety, stress, and anger can affect not only our health but our judgment and attention. Research has shown an effective way to deal with these difficult feelings: practicing mindfulness. Mindfulness allows us to pay attention to how we are thinking and feeling in the present moment, without judging whether the feelings are good or bad.

A basic method to cultivate mindfulness is to focus your attention on your breathing. This practice is simply called *mindful breathing*.[38] After setting time aside to practice mindful breathing, you should find it easier to refocus your attention on breathing during your normal daily routine to reduce stress during critical moments.

1. Find a comfortable seated position to relax yourself. You could be seated on a pillow on the floor, or in your favorite chair. Keep your back upright and comfortable. Hands should be resting wherever they are most relaxed.

2. Notice and relax your body. If your shoulders are tight, try dropping them. Notice the weight of your body. Let yourself relax as you notice the different sensations in each part of your body.

3. Focus on your breath. Feel the natural flow of your breath as it comes in through your nostrils and out from your mouth. Take breaths that aren't too long or short. Notice where you feel the breath in your body—the abdomen, chest, throat, mouth, and nose. One breath at a time. As one breath ends, the next begins.

4. As you are breathing, you may notice your mind beginning to wander. This is natural. Just acknowledge that your mind has wandered. If you begin to think about other things, it's okay. Gently redirect yourself back to the rhythm of your breathing.

5. Continue breathing mindfully for five or seven minutes. Notice your breath in silence. If your mind begins to wander, bring yourself back to the

thought of your breath.

6. After a few minutes, begin to bring your awareness back to your entire body. Let yourself relax even more deeply after you offer yourself recognition for completing this healthy practice.

MINDFULNESS MOVEMENT PRACTICE AND DAILY ACTIVITY

This direction of gentle movement during daily activities is an invitation to delve deeper into the life of the body. We must make strides to experience the mind and body as one and bring them together. As with all mindfulness practices, this movement practice is meant to focus our attention on our sensations and thoughts, from moment to moment.

The movements in this guided meditation are meant to be done during daily activities such as grooming, hygiene, laundry, cooking, leisure, typing, and yes, even toileting. This practice is not about judging our movements. Rather, it's about doing them to help connect us more closely to our body while we move.

Do not force movements; relax into them. Use your concern and knowledge of your own body and its limits to help guide you in your everyday movements. Imagine yourself performing movements in a mindful way. In the next example, you can see how one can be mindful even during a task like teeth brushing.

1. Begin in an alert position—sitting straight or standing, whatever position the activity calls for.

2. Notice how the chair or floor supports your body. Feel how gravity works against your body, and sense the areas of your body touching the floor or chair. Feel your feet touching the floor.

3. Bring your attention to notice your breath. With each breath, allow the floor or chair to receive more of your weight. Notice how your chest and abdomen rise and fall with each breath.

4. When you're ready, breathe in and imagine yourself preparing to carry out your activity—in this case, brushing your teeth. Notice your body's sensations as you walk to the sink. Notice any thoughts or emotions that may surface in the moment and let them be. Guide your attention back to the sensations of your body.

5. Next, step up to the sink mindfully. Bring a sense of novelty and curiosity toward the movement. Feel the pressure in your feet as you walk; feel your arms as they sway while you walk. Stand still at the sink with your arms at your sides. Notice any unnecessary tension and see if you can release that

tension by straightening your back or lowering your shoulders.

6. Notice any thoughts or feelings, and acknowledge them before you let them pass like clouds in the sky. Bring your hands up to the toothbrush as you experience the strength in your arms overcoming gravity. Hold the toothbrush in your hands as you observe its size, shape, and texture.

7. Now reach for toothpaste. Feel the tube, how it has been uniquely crushed. Unscrew the cap and feel the texture and pressure of the cap. Squeeze the toothpaste, feeling the muscles in your hands tighten and the sensation the bottle gives to your hands.

8. As you brush, feel the bristles on your gums and between your teeth. Acknowledge the arm and shoulder strength you are using. You may notice the scent of the toothpaste, but just notice it without judgment. Turn your focus to your body's position, movements, and feelings. Observe your feelings, and let them pass up into the clouds.

9. Next, feel the pressure of the faucet to start the water. Put your hands in the water and notice the body movements involved in this activity. As you rinse and clean, notice how your body feels after the experience of brushing your teeth. If it felt right, congratulate yourself for completing this activity with mindfulness toward your movements.

If you experienced any negative emotions during this task, take time to reflect on and evaluate the movement and find ways to avoid recreating the movement that caused pain or discomfort. By practicing, we are able to understand our bodies in a deeper, healthier, and holistic fashion, to make more conscious decisions for our health and well-being.

Mindfulness skills allow us the ability to work with pain and discomfort by becoming aware and understanding the difference between pain and suffering. Pain is the physical signal or sensation that signifies something is happening within your body. Suffering is the interpretation, or dwelling on the mental pain.

A patient of mine, Adam, didn't know the difference between pain and suffering. "It was a slow shift for me to understand the difference between pain and suffering. I constantly mentally resisted and ruminated about the pain in my lower back. After a few months, it was all I could think about. I became hypersensitive to my back pain, even more so after I stopped exercising.

"After I had been introduced to some mindfulness techniques, I was able to break the cycle of suffering through my own back pain. I was able to understand the similarities and differences between my physical and mental pain. Once I developed some clarity through mindfulness, I began making much more progress in my physical therapy treatments."

[33] Jon Kabat-Zinn, *Coming to Our Senses: Healing Ourselves and the World Through Mindfulness*, London: Piatkus, 2005.

[34] Pamela Richardson, Rochelle McLaughlin, "Chapter 7," in: Lorraine Williams Pedretti, ed., *Pedretti's Occupational Therapy: Practice Skills for Physical Dysfunction*, 8th ed., St. Louis: Elsevier, 2018.

[35] Fadel J. Zeidan, "Mindfulness meditation-based pain relief employs different neural mechanisms than placebo and sham mindfulness meditation-induced analgesia," *Neuroscience,* November 2015; Judith Turner, "Mindfulness-based stress reduction and cognitive-behavioral therapy for chronic low back pain: Similar effects on mindfulness, catastrophizing, self-efficacy, and acceptance in a randomized controlled trial," *Journal of Pain*, November 2016.

[36] Zeidan, "Mindfulness meditation-based pain relief: A mechanistic account," *The Annals of the New York Academy of Sciences*, June 2016.

[37] *Living Well*, "Mindfulness exercises: 6. Body scan https://www.livingwell.org.au/mindfulness-exercises-3/6-body-scan/.

[38] Diana Winston, "A 5-minute breathing meditation to cultivate mindfulness," *Mindful*, 26 February 2016, www.mindful.org/a-five-minute-breathing-meditation.

Chapter 13

Your Own Healing Power

Back pain healing starts with YOU.

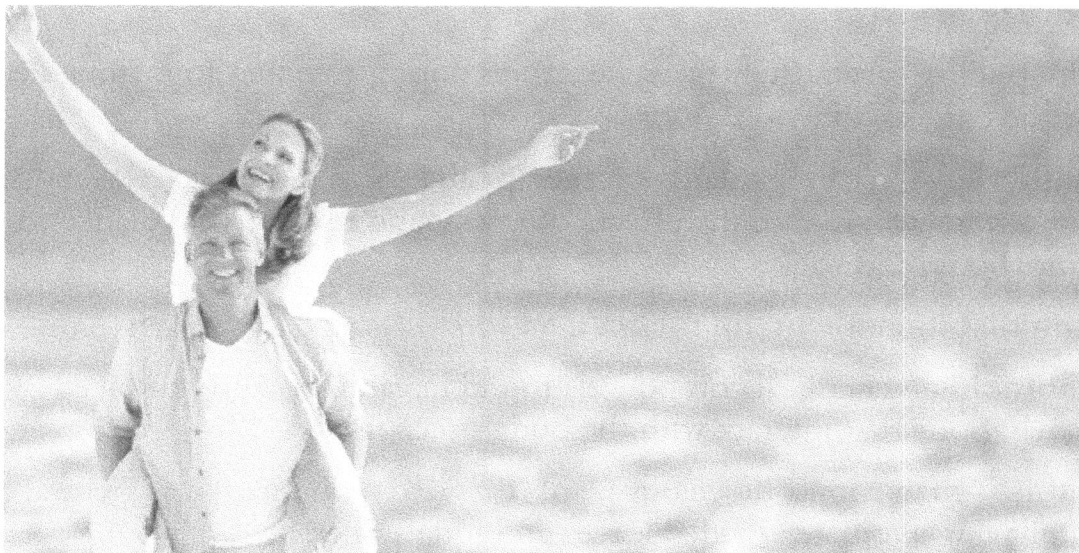

Everybody has energy and healing power. However, some people's healing powers have decreased. For example, a scrape may take longer to heal for some people than others. Often people no longer realize that they still have the ability within to reduce their pain.

I have shared with you some holistic solutions that have been effective for me and my clients. If you can remember to stay optimistic and embrace the fact that *YOU DO HAVE THE HEALING POWER*, your body will become better able to heal. You can begin to enjoy an active, pain-free lifestyle. However, remain cautious and sensible here, because you could actually hurt yourself. It is important to seek the guidance of a professional such as a caring and compassionate physical therapist, occupational therapist, doctor, chiropractor, nutritionist, or holistic healthcare practitioner who can empower you to become more active without causing yourself harm.

Glossary of Terms

Activities of daily living (ADLs)—daily activities used primarily by occupational therapists. ADLs include bathing, showering, toileting, dressing, swallowing, eating, feeding yourself, functional mobility, using personal devices, carrying out personal hygiene and grooming, and sexual activity.

Activity pacing—mindfully pacing exertion during activities to maintain energy for the entire activity.

Aromatherapy—a caring, hands-on therapy that aims to induce relaxation, increase energy, reduce the effects of stress, and restore lost balance to the mind, body, and soul.

Bulging disc—another term for *prolapsed vertebral disc.*

Cannabinoids—chemical compounds found in cannabis and produced by the human body that interact with the body's receptors.

Cannabis—a tall annual dioecious plant (*Cannabis sativa*) native to Central Asia and having alternate, divided leaves and tough fibers.

Carpal tunnel syndrome—a condition that causes pain, numbness, and tingling in the hand and arm. This condition occurs when the median nerve is squeezed or compressed as it travels through the wrist. Carpal tunnel syndrome usually stems from repetitive motions done at home or work.

Carrier oil—also known as a base or vegetable oil, a carrier oil is used to dilute essential oils before they are applied to the skin in massage and aromatherapy.

Cauda equina—the nerve roots in the lower end of the spinal cord.

Cauda equina syndrome—a dysfunction that occurs when the nerve roots of the cauda equina are compressed, usually from inflammation or compression, and they become unable to function. This can be the result of a herniated disc, fracture, tumor, trauma, or spinal stenosis. This can interrupt motor and sensory function to the lower extremities and bladder.

Chiropractor—a health professional concerned with the diagnosis, treatment, and prevention of mechanical disorders of the musculoskeletal system and the effects of these disorders on the function of the nervous system and general health. Chiropractors emphasize manual treatments, including spinal adjustment and other joint and soft-tissue manipulation.

Core—foundational musculature that provides support to the lower back and allows an individual to effectively and efficiently coordinate movement of their arms, legs, and spine.

C-reactive protein—plasma protein that rises in the blood as a result of inflammation from certain conditions.

Cryotherapy—use of cold as a medical treatment.

CT scan—a type of body imaging that produces many cross-sectional images using X-rays and a computer.

Degenerative discs—normal changes that take place in the discs of the spine, sometimes causing pain and stiffness.

Diffuser—device that disperses essential oils so their aroma fills a room or an area with natural fragrance.

Diode laser—laser diodes convert electrical energy to light.

Disc—found between one vertebra and its neighbors within the spine, discs are composed of two main parts: the annulus, comprising a series of leathery rings, and the nucleus, which is the jelly-like interior.

Disc herniation—occurs when a spinal disc protrudes through a crack, usually irritating nearby nerves.

Disc protrusion—occurs when the interior (nucleus) region of a vertebral disc protrudes, or extends past, the exterior (annulus) region of the vertebral disc.

Discogram—an invasive diagnostic test that uses X-rays to observe the intervertebral discs of the spine. A special dye is injected into the injured disc or series of discs. This dye makes the disc visible on a fluoroscope monitor and X-ray film.

Electromyography (EMG)—a procedure in which electrodes applied to the skin measure muscle response or electrical activity in response to a nerve's stimulation of the muscle.

Endocannabinoid deficiency syndrome—a condition in which a person produces reduced amounts of cannabinoids, which are considered to be essential in the promotion of health, vitality, and well-being.

Endocannabinoid receptors—a class of cell membrane receptors located throughout the body that are part of the endocannabinoid system, which is involved in a variety of physiological processes, including appetite, pain-sensation, mood, and memory.

Endocannabinoid system—a biological system composed of endocannabinoids and cannabinoid receptor proteins that are expressed throughout the central nervous system.

Endorphins—also known as the body's natural painkillers, endorphins bind chiefly to opiate receptors and produce some pharmacological effects (such as pain relief) in the same way that medicinal opiates do.

Energy (laser)—power absorbed by the body at a cellular level, from the utilization of physical or chemical resources.

Energy conservation—a way to perform activities that minimizes muscle fatigue, joint stress, and pain.

Epidural—a type of anesthesia that doctors administer to numb spinal nerves and prevent pain signals from traveling to the brain.

Ergonomic design—equipment and furniture design and body positioning with concern for efficiency, comfort, and prevention of injury in the home or working environment.

Facet injection—a minimally invasive procedure administered by a physician. It includes an injection of a small amount of local anesthetic and/or medication to numb a facet joint and provide pain relief.

Facet joint—a joint that allows the spine to bend and twist, and keeps the back from slipping too far forward or twisting without limits.

Facet joint syndrome—pain at the joint in between two vertebrae, often caused by osteoarthritis.

Gluteal muscles—the group of muscles that make up the buttocks. Used primarily for hip and leg extension.

Hamstrings—one or more of the three posterior thigh muscles in between the hip and the knee. The muscle group consists of the semimembranosus, semitendinosus, and biceps femoris muscles.

Hemp—the fiber of the cannabis plant, found in the stem and used to make rope, strong fabrics, fiberboard, and paper. Hemp contains less than 0.3 percent THC.

Herbs—plants with leaves, seeds, or flowers used for flavoring, food, medicine, or perfume.

Hip flexors—a group of muscles that makes up the front of the thigh. Used primarily for hip flexion.

Holistic—a system-wide approach that is concerned with complete systems rather than the analysis of, treatment of, or dissection of a system into parts. Holistic medicine attempts to treat both the mind and the body, the human and the environment, as a single system.

Impingement—also referred to as a *pinched nerve*, this occurs when inflammation surrounds a nerve and compresses it, causing pain.

Inflammation—the body's immune-system response to an irritant. This includes the release of antibodies and proteins delivered via the blood. The increased blood flow to the damaged area causes swelling.

Interleukin—a class of proteins produced by leukocytes (immune cells) for regulating immune responses.

Intracellular—located or occurring within a cell or cells.

ISO—isometric muscle contraction, which occurs without actual movement.

ISO-Abs—an isometric exercise engaging the abdominal muscles. It involves lying on the back with knees bent and feet flat on the floor.

Joint mobilization—the act of moving joints through their range of motion (ROM).

Kinesiology tape—a specific mode of treatment that involves placing strips of medical-grade, flexible tape on the body in specific directions to improve mobility and support joints, muscles, and tendons.

Laser power—the average laser power emission over time, expressed in mW.

Log roll—the act of rolling the body as one unit, without bending at the back, by leaning to one side while lying faceup, facedown, or sideways.

Long-arm reacher—a device with a claw arm and trigger used to access out-of-reach items.

Lumbago—a general diagnosis that can include conditions such as disc herniation, nerve impingement, spinal stenosis, and facet joint syndrome.

Lumbar vertebrae—area of the spinal column consisting of five individual cylindrical bones that form the spine below the rib-cage in the lower back. These vertebrae carry the upper body's weight while providing flexibility in movement to the trunk.

Macrophage—a type of white blood cell, of the immune system, that engulfs and digests cellular debris, foreign substances, microbes, and cancer cells.

Meditation—a technique for resting the mind and attaining a state of consciousness that is different from the normal waking state.

Micronutrients—the nutrients your body needs in the form of vitamins and minerals.

Mindfulness—the state of being conscious or aware.

Mitochondria—organelles in which the biochemical processes of respiration and energy production occur. Nicknamed the powerhouses of the cell, they are found in large numbers in most cells. Singular is *mitochondrion*.

ML830 laser—low-powered laser beams that produce non-thermal effects on human tissue to accelerate recovery time after injury. These types of injuries consist of damage to the deep, sensitive layers of tissue beneath the epidermis, including muscular, neural, lymphatic, and vascular tissues.

MRI (magnetic resonance imaging)—a test that uses magnets, radio waves, and a computer to take detailed pictures inside the body.

Musculoskeletal system—a combination of the muscular and skeletal systems of the body.

Musculoskeletal—concerning the joints, bones, muscles, ligaments, tendons, or bursas.

mW—milliwatts.

Myofascial pain syndrome—pressure on trigger points and muscular linings (fascia) that causes pain in the muscle and sometimes in unrelated parts of the body.

Neovascularization—the natural formation of new blood vessels.

Nerve root compression—occurs when herniated discs within the spine compress nerve roots, which may cause profound neurological damage, including motor and sensory loss.

Nervous system—tissues that record and distribute information within a person by means of electrical and chemical processes. The system comprises the brain, spinal cord, and nerves.

Neutral body position—when the joints are straight and the spine is aligned, not twisted.

Non-steroidal anti-inflammatory drugs (NSAIDs)—pain relief medicines such as ibuprofen. Available for purchase without a prescription, NSAIDs are one of the most common pain relief medicines in the world.

Nutrient—any substance that is absorbed by the body to provide energy, enable growth, and repair or perform proper functioning.

Occupational therapy—a type of therapy that helps people across the lifespan to do the things they want and need to do through the therapeutic use of daily activities and occupational activities.

Occupational therapists—medical professionals and assistants who help people participate in the things they want and need to do— such as dressing, bathing, leisure activity, and so on—through the therapeutic use of everyday activities (occupations).

Osteoporosis—a condition in which bone density decreases, causing bones to become weak and brittle.

Photoreceptors—a structure in a living organism, specifically a sensory cell or sense organ, that responds to light falling on it.

Physical therapy—method of treatment of disease, injury, or deformity by physical methods such as massage, physical modalities (heat, electric stimulation, etc.), and exercise rather than by drugs or surgery.

Physical therapists—trained and licensed medical professionals with experience in diagnosing physical abnormalities, restoring physical function and mobility, maintaining physical function, and promoting physical activity and proper function.

Prolapsed disc—when the annulus within a vertebral disc begins to break down and a resulting tear (or channel) causes the nucleus to bulge outside the disc.

Rehab facility—rehabilitation facilities can be inpatient or outpatient facilities that provide services to patients who are recovering from trauma or injury.

ROM—range of movement.

Sciatica—pain affecting the back, hip, and side of the leg. It is caused by compression of a spinal nerve root in the back, the sciatic nerve. It is often caused by degeneration of an intervertebral disc.

Selective nerve block—a medication, usually an anesthetic or anesthetic with steroid, that is administered near the spinal nerve where it exits the intervertebral foramen (the bony opening between adjacent vertebrae). This procedure reduces inflammation and numbs the pain transmitted by the nerve.

Sleep hygiene—sleep habits that relate to your ability to fall asleep and stay asleep.

Slipped disc—a vertebral disc that is displaced or protruding.

Sock aid—a device used to help put on socks without bending the back.

Soft tissue mobilization—a hands-on technique by a trained professional performed on muscles, ligaments, and fascia in order to break down adhesions and optimize muscle function.

Spinal stenosis—a condition that occurs when the spinal canal, which houses the spinal cord, becomes compressed or narrow. Compression of the spinal cord can cause pain and nerve irritation.

Spondylolisthesis—a displacement of a vertebra that sometimes occurs with the lower lumbar vertebrae. Vertebrae can slide out of alignment over time.

Synovial fluid—fluid found between and around joints. It lubricates the articular cartilages of synovial joints during movement.

Terpenes—organic compounds that provide aroma and flavor in plants and a variety of other organisms.

THC—tetrahydrocannabinol, a crystalline compound that is the main active ingredient in cannabis that produces psychoactive effects.

Trigger point—a hyperirritable spot; a palpable nodule in the taut bands of skeletal muscles. Also known as a *myofascial trigger point* or malfunctioning muscle tissue.

Trigger point release—the manual release of a tight area within muscle tissue that is causing pain in other parts of the body.

Wavelength—the distance between the crest of each wave, measured in nanometers (nm), where 1 nm is a billionth of one meter. This measurement is used specifically for cold laser treatment. Certain wavelengths have a greater effect on cellular activity.

www.ingramcontent.com/pod-product-compliance
Lightning Source LLC
Chambersburg PA
CBHW080625030426
42336CB00018B/3080